# INMAN'S JOINTS OF THE ANKLE

*SECOND EDITION*

# INMAN'S
# JOINTS
## *of the*
# ANKLE

*SECOND EDITION*

*Edited by*

## JAMES B. STIEHL, M.D.

*Assistant Professor*
*Clinical Director of Orthopaedic Research*
*Department of Orthopaedic Surgery*
*Medical College of Wisconsin*
*Milwaukee, Wisconsin*

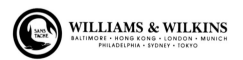

**WILLIAMS & WILKINS**
BALTIMORE · HONG KONG · LONDON · MUNICH
PHILADELPHIA · SYDNEY · TOKYO

*Editor:* Timothy H. Grayson
*Associate Editor:* Carol Eckhart
*Copy Editor:* Klementyna L. Bryte
*Designer:* Dan Pfisterer
*Illustration Planner:* Lorraine Wrzosek
*Production Coordinator:* Charles E. Zeller

*Printed in the United States of America*

First Edition 1976

**Library of Congress Cataloging-in-Publication Data**

Inman's joints of the ankle. — 2nd ed.   /   [edited by] James B. Stiehl.
　　　p.　　cm.
　　Rev. ed. of: The joints of the ankle  /  Verne T. Inman. c1976.
　　Includes bibliographical references and index.
　　ISBN 0-683-07976-X
　　1. Ankle.　I.　Stiehl, James B.　　II.　Inman, Verne Thompson, 1905–1980
Joints of the ankle.　　III.　Title: Joints of the ankle.
　　[DNLM: 1.　Ankle Joint.　　WE 880 1571]
QM549.I55　　1991
611'.718 — dc20
DNLM/DLC
for Library of Congress　　　　　　　　　　　　　　　　90-13096
　　　　　　　　　　　　　　　　　　　　　　　　　　　　CIP
　　　　　　　　　　　　　　　　　　　　　　　91 92 93 94
　　　　　　　　　　　　　　　　　　1 2 3 4 5 6 7 8 9 10

## In Memoriam

Verne T. Inman, M.D., Ph.D., was Professor and former Chairman of the Department of Orthopaedic Surgery at the University of California, San Francisco. He was Director of the Biomechanics Laboratory at the same institution from 1957 to 1973. Throughout his distinguished career, he wrote authoritatively about biomechanical subjects and was one of the pioneers in the use of electromyography in the analysis of muscle function. The first edition of *The Joints of the Ankle* detailed his meticulous morphologic and biomechanical studies of the talocrural joint, the tibiofibular syndesmosis and the subtalar joint. His concepts and conclusions have stood the test of time and anyone interested in this field would recognize the magnitude and impact of his work.

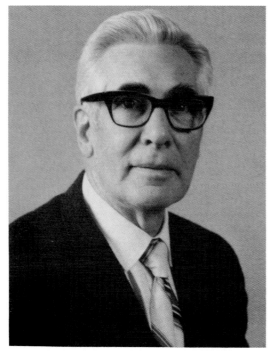

VERNE T. INMAN, M.D., Ph.D.
1905–1980

*Dedicated to My Wife,*
*Martha,*
*for her unwavering support,*
*and my children,*
*Amanda, Kurt and Henry*

# Foreword

It has been 15 years since the late Verne T. Inman (1905–1980) published his classic monographic entitled "The Joints of the Ankle." Dr. Inman, an orthopaedic surgeon with a Ph.D. in anatomy, possessed the ability to study an anatomical problem and ingeniously create models (which he built himself) to demonstrate joint function. Within this text the reader observes how the scientific method is applied step by step to first dissect and then reconstruct into a functioning unit "The Joints of the Ankle."

The information contained in this monograph must be studied on more than one occasion to gain a complete understanding of the coordinated events that occur about the ankle, subtalar, and transverse tarsal joints. Only through a thorough understanding of the function of the foot and ankle complex is the orthopaedic surgeon able to gain further insight into the multitude of clinical conditions presented to us.

In reviewing this monograph, Dr. Stiehl and his coauthors have retained much of the basic material and models created by Dr. Inman, which permit the reader to see how his conclusions were reached. At the same time they have brought many of the concepts presented in the original monograph up to date with supporting data from the current literature. It is interesting to note how the current literature has helped to reinforce most of the original concepts, rather than change them. A section describing the clinical relevance of the material has been added to the end of each chapter, which enhances understanding of the material. Many times, early in one's career, when so many new ideas and concepts are being formulated within one's mind, one cannot quite grasp the relevance of experimental or theoretical concepts, and this statement of clinical relevance is very useful.

It is a distinct privilege to have worked with Dr. Inman in his biomechanics lab during part of my orthopaedic career while director of the Gait Analysis Laboratory at the Shriner's Hospital in San Francisco. He was a brilliant man who truly had the ability to present original thoughts regarding the biomechanics of gait, the joints of the ankle, and most of the musculoskeletal system. I am pleased that we have an updated version of "The Joints of the Ankle" for those who want to acquire insight into the scientific methodology and its clinical relevance.

Roger A. Mann, M.D.
Oakland, California

# Preface

The magic of a classic textbook comes from the reader's insight regarding the author's descriptions and ideas. It is no different with the enjoyment of classical music or a fine old movie. Inman had devoted much of his professional career to morphologic and gait studies of the foot and ankle joints. It can be stated that countless readers have spent leisure hours absorbing the material that was presented in the original edition of *The Joints of the Ankle*. The editor and contributors to this subsequent edition have attempted to preserve much of the information as it existed in the initial text, recognizing that our own research and knowledge of recent developments have filled some of the gaps. It is apparent that little if any of Inman's own research efforts and conclusions have been questioned or modified in this edition. Inman did, however, offer opinions regarding topics that he had reviewed in the literature and speculated on their scientific significance. That purpose ultimately has lead to this revision; we have taken almost 15 years of new developments and incorporated them, correcting and deleting much, as Inman had done. As textbooks go, this really is a new book, but a firm foundation was laid by Dr. Inman. Only time will tell if we have maintained the "tradition."

J.B.S.

# Contributors

GERALD F. HARRIS, Ph.D.
*Associate Professor of Biomedical Engineering and Orthopaedic Surgery*
*Department of Orthopaedic Surgery*
*Medical College of Wisconsin and Marquette University*
*Milwaukee, Wisconsin*

JEFFREY E. JOHNSON, M.D.
*Assistant Professor*
*Department of Orthopaedic Surgery*
*Medical College of Wisconsin*
*Milwaukee, Wisconsin*

ARSEN M. PANKOVICH, M.D.
*Booth Memorial Hospital*
*Flushing, New York*

BRUCE J. SANGEORZAN, M.D.
*Department of Orthopaedic Surgery*
*University of Washington Medical School*
*Seattle, Washington*

JAMES B. STIEHL, M.D.
*Assistant Professor*
*Clinical Director of Orthopaedic Research*
*Department of Orthopaedic Surgery*
*Medical College of Wisconsin*
*Milwaukee, Wisconsin*

# Contents

---

### CHAPTERS

---

## APPENDICES

# 1

# Anthropomorphic Studies
# of the Ankle Joint

### JAMES B. STIEHL, M.D.

## WEDGE SHAPE OF THE TROCHLEA OF THE TALUS

The trochlea of the talus is generally considered to be wider anteriorly than posteriorly. Without exception, all texts of anatomy state clearly that the trochlea, when
viewed from above, is wedge shaped and the mediolateral dimension is greater anteriorly than posteriorly (2, 4–7).

A few texts provide actual measurements for the difference in the transverse width
of the trochlea. Frazer (3) stated that the trochlea is about 4 mm wider in front than
behind. Humphrey (8) and Piersol (15) reported that the trochlea is about one-fourth
narrower behind than in front. Luschka (12) stated that the posterior end is about
one-sixth narrower than is the opposite end. Macalister (13) stated that the posterior
width is four-fifths of the anterior width. Testut and Latarjet (17) reported an anterior
width that is from 5 to 6 mm greater than is the posterior.

Individual articles that discuss the "wedging" of the trochlea also reveal similar
discrepancies. Sewell, in an exhaustive study (16) of over 1000 Egyptian skeletons
from the Fifth Dynasty to the Roman period, reported that the average ratio of the
anterior transverse dimension of the trochlea to the posterior transverse width is 1:0.8,
with a range of 1:0.7 to 1:0.9. Barnett and Napier (1) investigated 152 cadaver tali
and found considerable variation in individual tali, some showing marked and others
minimal wedging. The implication of this variability is that some tali may show
parallelism of the medial and lateral facets whereas others show significant posterior
convergence.

Inman (9) confirmed the above findings when he measured the average difference
in anterior and posterior width on 100 specimens. The average posterior width of
the talus was less than the anterior width by 2.4 ± 1.3 mm, with a range of 0 to 6
mm (Fig. 1.1) (see Appendix B). Inman concluded from literature review and his own
cadaver tali measurements that the difference in anterior and posterior transverse
dimension ranged from 0 to 6 mm. In a small number of specimens (less than 5%),
the sides of the trochlea are essentially parallel with no wedging. The vast majority
demonstrated significant wedging, some as much as 25% difference.

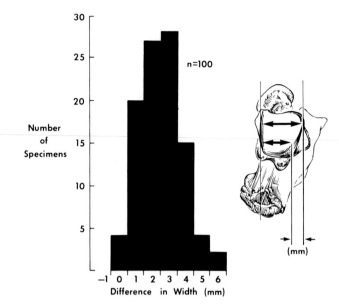

**Figure 1.1.** Histogram showing distribution of differences in width of 100 cadaver tali. The measurements were made in a plane perpendicular to the surface of the tibial facet.

## AMOUNT OF POSTERIOR CONVERGENCE OF MALLEOLAR FACETS

Consideration of the wedge shape of the trochlea of the talus in the transverse plane immediately raises the question of whether the malleolar facets are oriented to parallel the corresponding articular surfaces on the medial and lateral sides of the trochlea. If so, the planes of the malleolar facets should also converge posteriorly. Inman dissected one hundred cadaver ankle joints and in all cases found contiguous articular surfaces between malleolar and talar facets. Furthermore, the malleolar and talar facets appeared to remain in contact throughout the entire range of motion.

To confirm this later finding, he compared the angles of convergence between the planes of the facets on each talus and on the corresponding cast of the interior of each mortise (see Appendix A). On each specimen, the angle of posterior convergence of the facets of the talus and the corresponding angle of the malleolar facets were found to be identical. Further confirmation of the constant articulation of the ankle joint was suggested by McCullough and Burge (14) and Libotte et al. (10), who independently studied this phenomenon using the injection of dye to study contact areas. Both authors have concluded that a noticeable increase in contact occurs in weight bearing, and the trochlea of the talus is in contact with the medial malleolus and fibula through all positions of motion. Lindsjo et al. (11) used transverse computer tomography to study the ankle joint and found as well that the perfect fit of the talar trochlea between the malleoli is seen in all images. This occurred from full plantar flexion to dorsiflexion.

## CURVATURE OF THE TROCHLEA AS MEASURED ON ITS MEDIAL AND LATERAL SIDES

Inman (9) investigated the anatomical curvature of the talus by first determining the relationship of the verticle plane of each facet to the empirical axis of the ankle joint. Subsequently, the curvature of each facet was determined. The empirical axis of the ankle of 104 cadaver ankles was located using a previously described optical technique, and a 3-mm stainless steel rod was passed through this axis. As will be discussed in a later chapter, there is no single rigid axis of the ankle joint, but for the purpose of this study, the technique was deemed adequate (see Appendix A).

The angle between the vertical plane of the lateral talar facet and the ankle axis was 89.2 ± 2.8° with a range of 80–95°. The vertical plane of the medial facet compared to the ankle axis made an angle of 83.9 ± 5.2° with a range of 70–93° (Fig. 1.2) (see Appendix C). We see that the average angles of the two facets, when compared to the ankle joint axis and the distribution curves for the angles of each facet, were distinctly different. The vertical plane of the lateral talar facet always lay close to being perpendicular to the ankle joint axis. The variation of angular values for this relationship was very narrow with a standard deviation of 2.8°. The vertical plane of the medial talar facet was always oblique to the axis of the ankle joint and had considerably more variation with a standard deviation of 5.2°.

Inman used three independent techniques to calculate the curvature of each talar facet: a specially built contourometer, a Formagage, and a modified precision divider (see Appendix D). Inman found that the lateral talar facet approximated an arc of a circle in virtually all cases. On the medial side, when the arc of the medial talar facet was contoured into the plane of the axis of the ankle joint, 80% of the tali (86 of

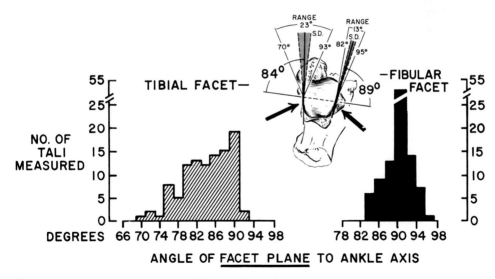

**Figure 1.2.** Angle of orientation of tibial and fibular facets to empirical axis of ankle joint. The histograms depict the distributions of the values from 104 cadaver tali.

107) described an arc of a circle. In the other 20% (21 of 107), this arc deviated to a varying extent from a circle. The reason for this later noncircularity is not fully understood but may relate in some degree to the fact that the axis of the ankle joint moves from plantar flexion to dorsiflexion.

Barnett and Napier (1) postulated that two different curvatures of arc may occur about the medial talar facet. Thus, they suggested a "dorsiflexion" axis that defined the ankle joint axis from midposition to full dorsiflexion and a "plantar flexion" axis from midposition to full plantar flexion. Another interesting observation made by these authors is the noncircularity of the medial talar facet in the vertical plane of the medial talar facet. This can be explained by the obliquity of this plane to the axis of the ankle joint if the vertical plane perpendicular to the ankle joint usually describes a circle.

Inman determined the curvature of the 86 tali where circularity was found on the medial talar facet. When comparing the radius curvature, in no specimen was the medial greater than the lateral radius. The average difference between the medial and lateral sides of the trochlea was 2.1 ± 1.1 mm, with a range of 0–6 mm (1). Inman then determined the amount of articular surface on the medial and lateral facets by dropping radii from the farthest extent of the radius of curvature to the center of curvature. Chords or straight lines were then drawn connecting the inter-section points of the anterior and posterior radii with the arc of curvature. The length of the chord was used to measure and compare the extent of articular cartilage on the medial and lateral sides of the trochlea. The average length of the chords was found to be 21.4 ± 4.5 mm on the lateral side and 16.4 ± 3.8 mm on the medial

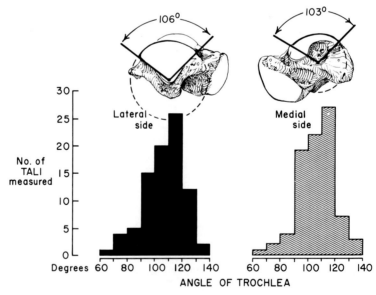

**Figure 1.3.** Average angles, almost identical, subtended by arcs of curvature of trochlea on lateral and medial sides. Note that the distributions of the individual values as shown in the histograms are also similar.

side, indicating the average exposed articular cartilage was greater on the lateral side than on the medial side. The angle subtended by the two radii on the medial and lateral sides, however, was almost identical, measuring 106 ± 13° on the lateral side and 103 ± 14° on the medial side (Fig. 1.3).

## COMPARISON OF ARCS OF THE FACETS WITH THOSE OF THE MALLEOLI

Inman performed an identical study of the mortise of each talus to determine the anatomical fit of each talus. This was done using dental stone casts of each mortise (see Appendix A). Using the same techniques outlined above, Inman determined the arc of curvature, the radii of curvature of the corresponding medial and lateral sides, and the anteroposterior dimensions of the medial and lateral sides by measuring chords.

The contour tracing of both malleolar facets from the mortises of 107 ankles (see Appendix D) could in all instances be fitted to the arcs of circles. On the lateral side, the arcs subtended an angle of 69 ± 8°. In all specimens, the lateral side of the plafond was found to be circular. The length of the arc of curvature of the medial side was always shorter than the lateral side. The average subtended angle was 55 ± 11°. Several of the medial tracings were very short subtending angles less than 40°. Therefore, in about 15% of the casts, is was impossible to state with certainty that the medial side was truly circular.

The radii of the arcs of curvature of each trochlea and corresponding mortise were compared for accuracy of fit on both the medial and lateral sides of the joint. On the lateral (fibular) side, the average lengths of radii of curvature were found to be nearly the same within 1 mm. When specific data were reviewed, 30% (26 of 86) of the trochlea and corresponding mortises were identical. In the remainder, the radius of the trochlea was either 1 mm greater or less than the mortise. In nine specimens, the mortise was 2 mm greater than the trochlea. Inman stated that this technique was not adequate to detect differences less than 1 mm. From this data, he concluded that the fit on the lateral side of the joint must be a close one.

On the medial (tibial) side, the difference in the measured radii of the trochlea and mortises was greater. The average difference was 2.1 ± 1.1 mm, with a range of 0–5 mm. The radius of curvature of the mortise on the medial side was greater than its corresponding trochlea in all specimens.

Inman concluded that the talus fits snugly in the mortise on the lateral side but rather loosely on the medial side. A few millimeters of anteroposterior play on the medial side of the ankle joint appears to be possible. Furthermore, this motion could account for several degrees of horizontal rotation of the talus within the mortise. This anatomical fact will gain relevance in our subsequent discussion of the shifting axis of the ankle joint.

### References

1. Barnett CH, Napier JR. The axis of rotation at the ankle joint in man: Its influence upon the form of the talus and mobility of the fibula. J Anat 1952;86:1.
2. Cunningham DJ. Cunningham's textbook of anatomy. 10th ed. Roamanes GJ, ed. London: Oxford University Press, 1964.
3. Frazer JE. The anatomy of the human skeleton. London: J and A Churchill, 1933.
4. Gardner E, Gray DJ, O'Rahilly R. Anatomy:

A regional study of human structure. 3rd ed. Philadelphia: WB Saunders, 1969.

5. Grant JCB. Grant's method of anatomy: By regions, descriptive and deductive. 8th ed. Basmajian JV, ed. Baltimore: Williams & Wilkins, 1971.

6. Gray H. Anatomy of the human body. 29th ed. Goss CM, ed. Philadelphia: Lea & Febiger, 1973.

7. Horner WE. A treatise on special and general anatomy. 4th ed. Philadelphia: Carey, Lea, and Blanchard, 1836.

8. Humphrey GM. A treatise on the human skeleton (including the joints). Cambridge: Macmillan and Co, 1858.

9. Inman VT. The joints of the ankle. Baltimore: Williams & Wilkins, 1976.

10. Libotte M, Klein P, Colpaert H, Alameh M, Plaimont P, Halleux P. Contribution a l'etude biomecanique de la pince malleolaire. Rev Chir Orthop 1982;68:299–305.

11. Lindsjo U, Hemmingsson A, Sahlstedt B, Danckwardt-Lilliestrom G. Computed tomography of the ankle. Acta Orthop Scand 1979;50:797–801.

12. Luschka H. von. Die anatomie der glieder des menschen. vol. 3, part 1. Tubingen: Verlap der Lauppschen Buchhandlung, 1865.

13. Macalister A. A text-book of human anatomy: Systematic and topographical, including the embryology, histology and morphology of man. Philadelphia: P. Blakiston, Son and Co., 1889.

14. McCullough CJ, Burge PD. Rotatory stability of the load-bearing ankle. J Bone Joint Surg 1980;62B:460–464.

15. Piersol GA, ed. Human anatomy, including structure and development and practical considerations. Philadelphia: JB Lippincott, 1907.

16. Sewell RBS. A study of the *Astragalus*. J Anat Physiol 1904;38:233.

17. Testut L, Latarjet A. Traite d'anatomie humaine. vol. 1 9th ed. Latarjet A, ed. Paris: G. Doin et Cie, 1948.

# 2

# Functional Morphology of the Trochlea

JEFFREY E. JOHNSON, M.D.

Based on the observations and data presented thus far, it is possible to postulate the following hypothesis: The trochlea of the talus is rarely, if ever, a section of a cylinder, but is a section of a frustum of a cone whose apex is directed medially and whose apical angle varies considerably from individual to individual. Support for this hypothesis can be deduced from the presently available data as summarized in Chapter 1. The greater anteroposterior dimensions of the lateral facet and of the articular cartilage on the lateral side of the trochlea compared with the medial side are suggestive of a cone. The radius of curvature is smaller on the medial side than the lateral side of the trochlea, which can be true only in a cone as opposed to a cylinder. The greater anteroposterior width of the plafond on the lateral side, as compared to the medial side, is in accord with the concept of a conical surface. Finally, Clark (2) demonstrated that soft wax, when molded over the trochlea and carefully flattened, produced the shape of a curved ribbon rather than a straight one. This could result only from molding over a conical surface rather than over a cylindrical surface.

Visual confirmation of the conical surface of the talus is graphically illustrated by rotating the talus within the mortise and making saw cuts at intervals into the trochlea as the talus is moved from full plantar flexion to full dorsiflexion. This was originally done by Close and Inman (3) on a few cadaver ankles and then repeated by Inman (5) in 86 cadaver specimens using a specially built holder and guide (see Appendix E). Each specimen was rotated in the holding jig about a fixed "empirical" axis of rotation, as determined by the author.

The converging saw cuts in four selected tali and the casts of their mortises are seen in Figure 2.1. When Kirschner wires are pressed into the saw cuts in each specimen, they converge toward the axis rod on the medial side of the talus (Figs. 2.2 and 2.3). The converging wires outline the shape of a cone, of which each trochlea is the frustum.

The average conical angle of the saw cuts on the 86 tali was $24 \pm 6°$ and on the cast of the mortise was $22 \pm 4°$. The distribution of the individual values of the apical angles is depicted in the histograms (Fig. 2.4). There was significant individual variation in the measured apical angles (range $0-38°$) with a few of the trochlea resembling a cylinder rather than a cone (5).

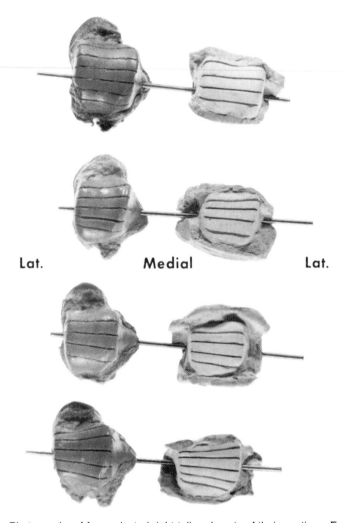

Lat.                    Medial                    Lat.

**Figure 2.1.**  Photographs of four selected right tali and casts of their mortises. Each talus with its cast is mounted on a single 3-mm stainless steel rod, which represents the estimated axis of rotation. Note the variation in the degree of convergence of the saw cuts. In the *top* photograph, the saw cuts are almost parallel, indicating that the trochlea approaches a section of a cylinder, and its cast shows that the mortise is quadrilateral in shape. The *bottom* photograph shows marked convergence of the saw cuts, and the cast shows the mortise to be trapezoidal.

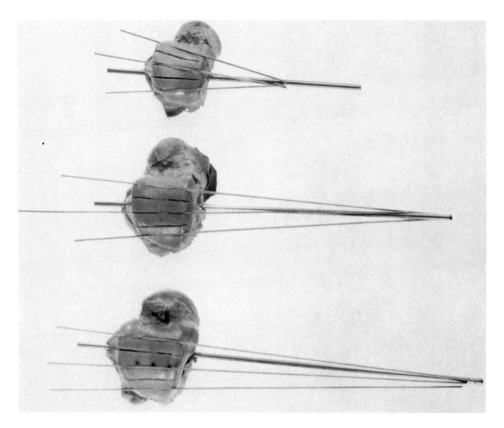

**Figure 2.2.** Photographs of three selected left tali viewed from above. Kirschner wires have been pressed into the saw cuts. Note their convergence onto the stainless steel rod representing the estimated axis of rotation.

The following facts concerning the talus have thus far been presented:

1. The radius of curvature of the trochlea is less on the medial than on the lateral side.
2. The arcs of curvature of the trochlear articular surfaces, although different, subtend the same angle.
3. Saw cuts in the trochlea made about a fixed axis converge toward the medial side.

Taken together, these facts confirm the basic concept that the trochlea is rarely a section of a cylinder, as some have previously stated, but rather a frustum of a cone, whose apical angle shows considerable individual variation (5).

The concept that the trochlea is a section of a frustum of a cone appears to explain some of the anatomic features of the ankle joint. The anteroposterior lengths of the articular facets on the two sides of the trochlea differ. The tibial facet is usually small, short, and comma-shaped and often terminates short of the posterior limits of the articular cartilage on the superior surface of the trochlea. The fibular facet is

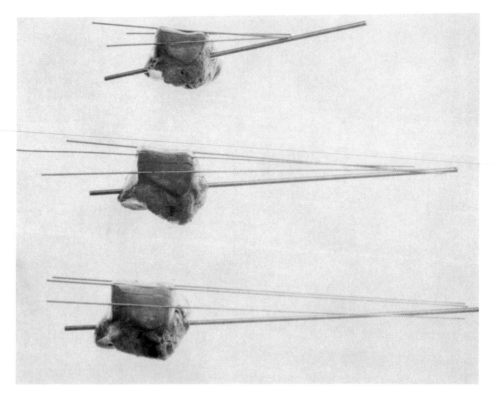

**Figure 2.3.** Same specimen as in Figure 2.2, viewed from the back. Note that the Kirschner wires outline half of a cone, with the rod representing the ankle axis corresponding to the axis of the cone. The obliquity of the ankle axis varies in the three tali and bears no relationship to the superior articular surface of the trochlea.

longer and always extends the entire length of the articular surface. This is exactly the situation one would expect to find if the trochlea were a frustum of a cone. Since the medial malleolus lies closer to the apex of the cone, for the same angular motion of the ankle, it would have less anteroposterior displacement than the base of the lateral malleolus, which lies farther from the apex. Figure 2.5 pictorially summarizes the concept of the morphology of the trochlea as a frustum of a cone (5).

It has been shown by Barnett and Napier (1), Hicks (4), and more recently by Sammarco (7), Siegler et al. (8) and Lundberg et al. (6) that the axis of rotation of the talus within the mortise is not about a fixed axis. Rather, it rotates about a variable axis in all three planes (dorsi-plantar flexion, inversion-eversion, and internal-external rotation). Despite Inman's assumption of a fixed axis of rotation, the facts confirming the conical shape of the trochlea should still be valid. Beginning from the assumption that the trochlea is conical rather than cylindrical in shape, certain anatomic facts about the ankle can be reevaluated.

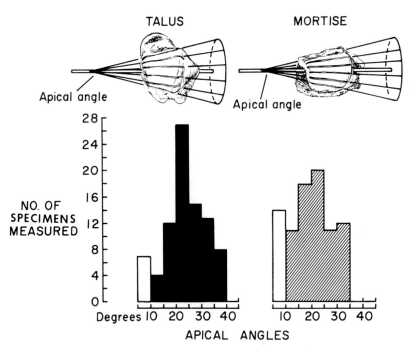

**Figure 2.4.** Variations in apical angles of conical surfaces of trochleas and casts of mortises. Angles were obtained by extrapolating from the end of the saw cuts toward the medial sides. All specimens whose apical angles were 10° or less were lumped together and are shown in the *clear bars* of the histograms.

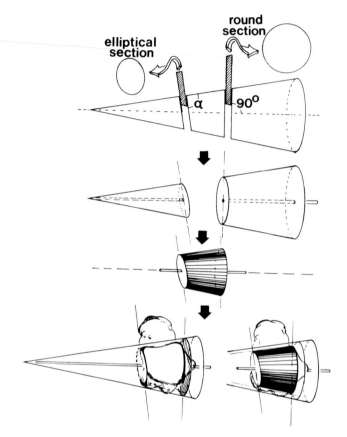

**Figure 2.5.** Pictorial representation of the concept that the trochlea of the talus is a section, or frustum, of a cone. The section of the cone cut at 90° to the axis of the cone is circular when projected onto a transverse plane of the cone and corresponds to the lateral (fibular) facet of the talus. The section cut obliquely is elliptical and corresponds to the medial (tibial) facet. Note that the fibular facet, being farther from the apex of the cone, possesses greater dimensions. With minor modifications, a section of the frustum is converted into the trochlea of the talus. The anteroposterior curve of the fibular facet is an ellipse because of the oblique orientation of the conical surface of the trochlea when viewed from above.

## References

1. Barnett CH, Napier JR. The axis of rotation at the ankle joint in man: Its influence upon the form of the talus and the mobility of the fibula. J Anat 1952;86:1.

2. Clark AE. The ankle joint of man [M.D. Thesis]. Berne: University of Berne, 1877.

3. Close JR, Inman VT. The action of the ankle joint. Prosthetic Devices Research Project, Institute of Engineering Research, University of California, Berkeley. Series 11, issue 22. The Project, Berkeley, 1952.

4. Hicks JH. The mechanics of the foot. I. The joints. J Anat 1953;87:345.

5. Inman VT. The joints of the ankle. Baltimore: Williams & Wilkins, 1976.

6. Lundberg A, Svensson OK, Nemeth G, Selvik G. The axis of rotation of the ankle joint. J Bone Joint Surg 1989;71B:94–99.

7. Sammarco J. Biomechanics of the ankle: Surface velocity and instant center of rotation in the sagittal plane. Am J Sports Med 1977;5(6):231–234.

8. Siegler S, Chen J, Schneck CD. The three dimensional kinematics and flexibility characteristics of the human ankle and subtalar joints. Part I: Kinematics. J Biomech Eng 1988;110:364–373.

# 3

# Shape of the Trochlea and Mobility of the Lateral Malleolus

JEFFREY E. JOHNSON, M.D.

Investigators prior to Inman (9) appear to have measured the transverse width of the trochlea in planes perpendicular to the tibial facet. For the study of the isolated talus, this seemed to be the most logical procedure, since the tibial articular facet appears parallel to the long axis of the bone. The tibial articular facet presents a flatter surface than that of the fibular facet and therefore could be employed as a reference plane. However, the angle between the plane of the tibial facet and the functional axis of the ankle has been shown to vary considerably from specimen to specimen. Therefore, it appears more reasonable to measure the width of each trochlea in relation to the functional transverse axis of the ankle. Using the saw cuts (see Fig. 2.1) as directional guides, the measurements are oriented along the conical surface of the trochlea.

When these measurements were made by Inman (9), as illustrated in Appendix E, the gross variation in the widths of the trochlea reported in previous studies seemed to disappear. In all specimens the differences in the widths from the most anterior to the most posterior saw cut were reduced to zero or at least were halved (i.e., difference was less than 2 mm). If the most anterior saw cut was compared with the center cut, the difference in width in any one specimen was negligible (within the limits of accuracy of measurement, or ± 1 mm). The same results were obtained when the middle saw cut width was compared with the most posterior cut.

This observation is further substantiated by the fact that when the distal tibio-fibular syndesmosis is rigidly fixed to prevent mortise widening with ankle motion, the degree of limitation of ankle dorsiflexion does not correlate with the difference in width of the anterior and posterior parts of the trochlea (20). If the trochlea were, in fact, "wedge" shaped, then one would expect a much stronger correlation (i.e., the trochlea with the greatest difference in anteroposterior width would have the greatest decrease in ankle dorsiflexion when the syndesmosis screw is inserted, and vice versa). However, this is not the case.

In any position, from full plantar flexion to full dorsiflexion, the articular surface of the distal tibia covers only one-half to two-thirds of the corresponding talar articular surface when viewed in the sagittal plane (3, 21). Knowing this, and that the difference

15

in measurement of the trochlea between the anterior width and the posterior width is small, it is understandable that a very small motion of the lateral malleolus is all that is theoretically required during movement of the talus in the mortise.

Actual measurements of the motion of the lateral malleolus with flexion and extension of the talus in the mortise have been made by several investigators (1, 3, 4, 7, 10, 11, 22). Despite the different methods used for measurement, lateral translation of the malleolus along the transverse axis has been reported to be 1.0–2.0 mm when the talus moves from maximum plantar flexion to maximum dorsiflexion. Karrholm et al. (11) showed that the greatest increase in width of the ankle mortise (averaging 1.2 mm) occurred when the ankle is moved from plantar flexion to the neutral position. Similar measurements were also made by Close and Inman (4) and Grath (7). However, the largest width of the ankle mortise (lateral malleolar displacement) occurred in most patients when the foot was maximally dorsiflexed (11). Therefore, it appears from both the direct measurements of trochlear width and direct measurements of the change in ankle mortise width with ankle flexion and extension, that less than 2.0 mm of lateral displacement of the distal fibula is all that is required to accommodate the most extremely wedge-shaped talus.

## CONCEPT OF THREE-DIMENSIONAL LATERAL MALLEOLAR MOTION

Lateral malleolar motion with ankle flexion and extension occurs not only along the transverse axis (mediolateral displacement) but also along the longitudinal axis (proximal-distal displacement), the sagittal axis (anteroposterior displacement), and around the longitudinal axis of the fibula (internal-external rotation).

Malleolar motion in the longitudinal and sagittal axes was discussed by Close (3) and Inman (9) but was felt to be negligible and no direct measurements were made. Karrholm et al. (11) used a roentgen stereophotogrammetric analysis to measure translation of the distal fibula in all axes (transverse, sagittal, longitudinal). Slight distal displacement of the lateral malleolus (0.1–0.5 mm) was observed when the ankle was moved from full plantar flexion to full dorsiflexion, with variability among the specimens. In one specimen, a proximal displacement of 0.4 mm was observed when the ankle was moved from plantar flexion to the neutral position. Further dorsiflexion resulted in a distal displacement of about the same amount. All of these observations were on passive motions of the ankle in the unloaded state. Scranton et al. (22) studied fibular motion in the loaded, active state in five normal subjects. By comparison of radiographs taken in the nonweight-bearing and weight-bearing positions, when the fibula was actively loaded, it migrated distally. Distal migration of the fibula was explained by the active contraction of the peronei, tibialis posterior, and flexor hallucis longus muscles on the fibula and interosseous membrane.

Jend et al. (10) measured tibiofibular motion in 25 normal subjects by computed tomography in the loaded and unloaded state. From ankle dorsiflexion to plantar flexion, the unloaded fibula moved an average $1.1 \pm 0.4$ mm medially with an accompanying nonsignificant anterior shift and internal rotation. Application of a static axial load to the ankle did not alter these findings. There was significant individual variation among the subjects, especially in anteroposterior shift of the fibula during motion of the ankle joint from full dorsiflexion to full plantar flexion. Approximately one-third of the group (mostly females) exhibited a posterior shift of the fibula during this motion and two-thirds demonstrated an anterior shift. With a static load applied, most of the fibular shift in the posterior shift group was eliminated. Application of load in the other group did not increase the amount of anterior fibular shift during ankle motion (10).

Karrholm (11) showed fibular translation along the sagittal axis, but it was quite variable between the nine subjects tested. Some lateral malleoli displaced anteriorly and some posteriorly when the ankle was moved from plantar flexion to the neutral position. However, all but one subject exhibited posterior displacement of the lateral malleolus when the ankle was moved from the neutral to the dorsiflexed position. All nine of the subjects studied by Karrholm were less than 18 years of age and five had open epiphyses at the ankle, which may limit some extrapolation to the kinematics of the adult ankle. This also may explain some of the measurements that suggested deformation of the distal fibula with greater displacement of the tip of the lateral malleolus than the metaphysis. To the extent that deformation of the distal fibula occurs in the actively loaded adult ankle is unknown.

Rotatory motion of the lateral malleolus about the longitudinal axis of the fibula during ankle dorsiflexion and plantar flexion was observed by Barnett and Napier (2) and Close (3). Barnett and Napier measured this in one subject and found a 3° lateral rotation of the fibula relative to the tibia during forced dorsiflexion of the ankle. They thought the amount of fibular rotation may be related to the orientation of the surfaces of the proximal tibiofibular joint. Ogden (19) studied fibular motion fluoroscopically and stated that rotation of the proximal fibula with ankle dorsiflexion was more pronounced in subjects with a more horizontally oriented proximal tibiofibular joint. Ogden further suggested that the position of the knee and the tautness of the fibular collateral ligament and the biceps tendon may also modulate the amount of fibular motion. Close (3) showed 5–7° of lateral rotation of the fibula with an external rotation force and 1° of medial rotation of the fibula with an internal rotation force applied to the intact ankle, but did not measure fibular rotation with ankle dorsiflexion and plantar flexion. Jend et al. (10) cited a study by Henkemeyer (8) on 26 cadaver ankles, which demonstrated 3.7° of axial rotation of the distal fibula with dorsiflexion and plantar flexion of the ankle. Accurate quantitative measurements of the rotation of the fibula during plantar flexion and dorsiflexion of the ankle, with or without the influence of muscular action or load, have not been made. Despite this, it is a generally accepted observation that external rotation of the fibula with respect to the tibia occurs with motion of the ankle from plantar flexion to dorsiflexion.

Motion of the lateral malleolus has been shown to occur in the transverse, sagittal, and longitudinal planes, with rotation about a vertical axis and with slight bending of the distal fibula. These motions have a significant individual variation. Application of static loads seems to decrease fibular motion in the sagittal plane axis but does not alter motion in the transverse axis or rotation about the vertical axis. This motion may be only barely perceptible since the changes in the mortise with dorsiflexion and plantar flexion of the ankle require at most 1–2 mm to adjust to the width of the trochlea.

## CLINICAL RELEVANCE

Because of this seemingly small amount of fibular motion, Inman (9) suggested that rigid internal fixation of a diastasis of the syndesmosis should cause little disability. This was substantiated by the clinical experience of several authors (5, 6, 14, 17). However, Scranton et al. (22) reported three cases of posttraumatic distal tibiofibular synostosis that was associated with significant ankle pain. All three patients were relieved of their pain following excision of the synostosis, presumably because the normal motion between the tibia and fibula was restored.

Olerud (20) showed in cadaver specimens that ankle range of motion in dorsiflexion was limited if the syndesmotic screw was inserted with the foot in plantar flexion. This substantiated the generally held recommendation that the syndesmotic screw should be inserted with the ankle in dorsiflexion to minimize the risk of a limitation in motion.

McCullough and Burge (13) demonstrated that rigid fixation of the distal tibiofibular joint with a clamp prevents normal ankle motion. However, the clamp used produced compression across the syndesmosis, similar to a lag screw, as opposed to the recommendation of the Association for the Study of Internal Fixation (ASIF) (16) that the syndesmotic screw be placed as a neutralization screw.

Needleman et al. (18) studied the effect of the syndesmotic screw on ankle motion in eight cadaver specimens. There was a statistically significant decrease in tibiotalar external rotation after syndesmotic screw fixation using the ASIF technique (16), regardless of foot position or the amount of axial load applied. They concluded that the syndesmotic screw should be removed prior to the return to full activity. Leaving it in place was shown to contribute to abnormal ankle motion, which could result in local discomfort and possible fatigue fracture of the screw (18).

There is a great variation in the functional anatomy of the human ankle. Those persons who can tolerate the presence of the syndesmotic screw during full activity may have certain anatomic features that predispose to less fibular motion during ankle function (18). Those with a limited range of motion in dorsiflexion seem to have a greater demand for motion between the fibula and the tibia for normal joint function (20). Perhaps this subgroup of patients should have the syndesmosis screw removed to avoid a limitation in ankle joint function.

There is still controversy between those advocating leaving the syndesmotic screw in place (6) and those advocating removal (12, 15, 18), prior to return to full activity following ankle fracture. Until further study is done, this clinical question will remain unanswered.

### References

1. Ashhurst APC, Bromer RS. Classification and mechanism of fractures of the leg bones involving the ankle, based on a study of three hundred cases from the Episcopal Hospital: Anatomic and surgical study. Arch Surg 1922;4:51.

2. Barnett CH, Napier JR. The axis of rotation at the ankle joint in man: Its influence upon the form of the talus and the mobility of the fibula. J Anat 1952;86:1.

3. Close JR. Some applications of the functional anatomy of the ankle joint. J Bone Joint Surg 1956;38A:761.

4. Close JR, Inman VT. The action of the ankle joint. Prosthetic Devices Research Project, Institute of Engineering Research, University of

California, Berkeley. Series 11, issue 22. The Project, Berkeley, 1952.

5. Costigan PG. Treatment of true widening of ankle mortise. Can Med Assoc J 1953;69:310.

6. DeSouza LT, Gustilo RB, Meyer TS. Results of operative treatment of displaced external rotation-abduction fractures of the ankle. J Bone Joint Surg 1985;67A:1066–1074.

7. Grath GB. Widening of the ankle mortise: A clinical and experimental study. Acta Chir Scand 1960;(suppl 263).

8. Henkemeyer H, Pueschel R, Burri C. Experimentelle untersuchungen zur biomechanik der syndesmose. Langenbecks Arch Chir (Suppl) Chir Forum 369–371, 1975, as cited in: Jend HH, Ney R, Heller M. Evaluation of tibiofibular motion under load conditions by computed tomography. J Orthop Res 1985;3:418–423.

9. Inman VT. The joints of the ankle. Baltimore: Williams & Wilkins, 1976.

10. Jend HH, Ney R, Heller M. Evaluation of tibiofibular motion under load conditions by computed tomography. J Orthop Res 1985;3:418–423.

11. Karrholm J, Hansson LI, Selvik G. Mobility of the lateral malleolus. Acta Orthop Scand 1985;56:479–483.

12. Mast JW, Teipner WA. A reproducible approach to the internal fixation of adult ankle fractures: Rationale, technique and early results. Orthop Clin North Am 1980;11(3):661–679.

13. McCullough CJ, Burge PD. Rotatory stability of the load-bearing ankle. J Bone Joint Surg 1980;62B:460–464.

14. Meekison M. Ankle injuries. In: Thomson JEM, Edwards JW, eds. The American Academy of Orthopaedic Surgeons presents lectures on reconstruction surgery, selected from the instructional courses of the Twelfth Annual Assembly, Chicago, January 23–24. Ann Arbor, MI: [The Academy], 1944.

15. Morris M, Chandler RW. Fractures of the ankle. Techniques Orthop 1987;2(3):10–19.

16. Mueller ME, Algower M, Schneider R, Willenegger H. Malleolar fractures. In: Manual of internal fixation. Technique recommended by the AO Group. 2nd ed. New York: Springer-Verlag, 1979:296.

17. Mullins JFP, Sallis JG. Recurrent sprain of the ankle joint with diastasis. J Bone Joint Surg 1958;40B:270.

18. Needleman RL, Skrade DA, Stiehl JB. Effect of the syndesmotic screw on ankle motion. Foot Ankle 1989;10(1):17–24.

19. Ogden JA. The anatomy and function of the proximal tibiofibular joint. Clin Orthop 1974;101:186–191.

20. Olerud C. The effect of the syndesmotic screw on the extension capacity of the ankle joint. Arch Orthop Trauma Surg 1985;104:299–302.

21. Sarrafian SK. Anatomy of the foot and ankle. Philadelphia: JB Lippincott, 1983.

22. Scranton PE, McMaster JH, Kelly E. Dynamic fibular function. Clin Orthop 1981;118:76–81.

**4**

# Axis of Rotation of the Ankle

## JEFFREY E. JOHNSON, M.D.

When an isolated tibia or an anteroposterior roentgenogram of the ankle is examined, it appears that the articular surface of the tibia lies in a plane that is at nearly a right angle to the long axis of the bone. Isman and Inman (4) measured the angle between the midline of the tibia and the plane of the plafond of the tibia. Their method was indirect and its accuracy questionable. Inman (3) reinvestigated that initial series and additional specimens were measured with a more direct method (see Appendix A). In 107 cadaver specimens, the angle measured in the coronal plane on the medial side between the midline of the tibia and the surface of the plafond of the ankle (Fig. 4.1) was found to be 93.3 ± 3.2°, with a range of 88–100° (3).

Inman (3) measured the angle between the empirical axis of the ankle joint (see Appendix A) and the midline of the tibia in the same series of specimens to be 82.7 ± 3.7°, with a range of 74–94° (Fig. 4.2).

The average angular difference between the empirical axis and plane of the plafond of the tibia was found to be 11.3 ± 4.1°, with a range of 2–21° (3). This means that in all the specimens the empirical axis was oblique to the articular surface of the ankle joint. In most specimens, the empirical axis was found to pass slightly distal to the tips of both malleoli but had considerable individual variation. For clinical purposes one can press one finger under the tip of each malleolus (Fig. 4.3) or on an anteroposterior radiograph connect the distal ends of the two malleoli (Fig. 4.4) and determine with reasonable accuracy the inclination of the ankle axis as projected on the coronal plane.

When it is appreciated that the trochlea is a frustum of a cone rather than a cylinder, it becomes apparent how the obliquity of the ankle joint axis in the coronal plane can vary between individuals even though the articular surfaces of the ankle joint appear to lie in a plane perpendicular to the long axis of the leg (3) (see Fig. 2.3).

The method used by Inman (3) to determine the empirical ankle axis (see Appendix A) required the assumption that plantar flexion and dorsiflexion of the ankle occurred around a fixed axis. Barnett and Napier (1) and Hicks (2) found that the ankle joint used different axes for plantar flexion and dorsiflexion. Since the work of Inman (3), several investigators have demonstrated that the axis of rotation of the ankle is not

21

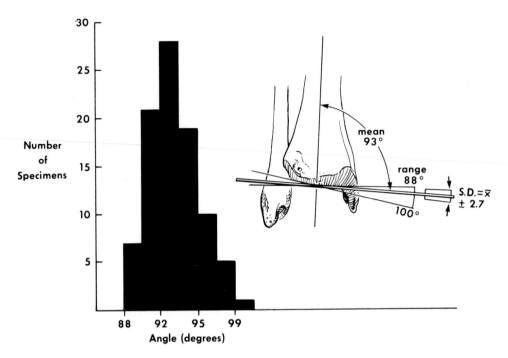

**Figure 4.1.** Variations in angle between the midline of tibia and plafond of mortise. The distribution of the values is shown in the histogram. Note the small amount of spread among the individual measurements (approximately 10°).

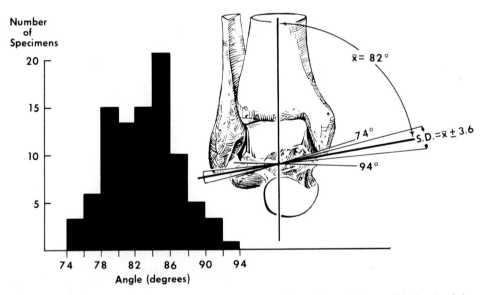

**Figure 4.2.** Variations in angle between the midline of the tibia and the empirical axis of the ankle. The histogram reveals a considerable spread of individual values.

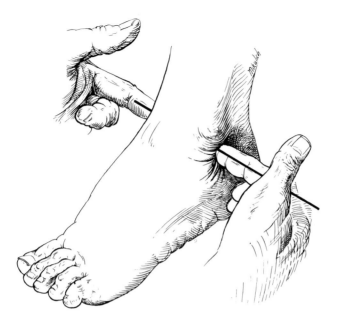

**Figure 4.3.** Estimation of position of ankle axis by palpation of malleoli. (From Inman VT, Mann RT. Biomechanics of the foot and ankle. In: Inman, VT ed. DuVries' surgery of the foot. 3rd ed. St. Louis: CV Mosby, 1973.)

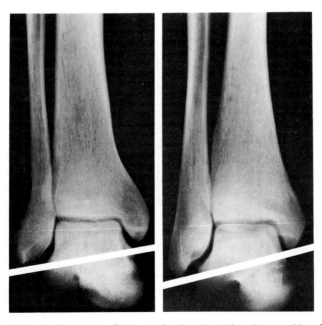

**Figure 4.4.** Anteroposterior x-rays of two randomly selected cadaver ankles. The rod representing the estimated axis of rotation passes just below the tips of the malleoli.

fixed but has a variable axis that changes continuously throughout the range of movement (5–8).

Lundberg et al. (6) analyzed the axis of rotation of the ankle joint by roentgen stereophotogrammetry in eight healthy volunteers in the weight-bearing position (Fig. 4.5). The individual discrete helical axes for each 10° of motion from 30° of plantar flexion to 30° of dorsiflexion were projected onto an outline of the ankle joint in both the coronal and horizontal planes (Figs. 4.6 and 4.7). From 30° of plantar flexion to 30° of dorsiflexion, the helical axis of the ankle joint, when projected onto a coronal plane, changed position from an inclination that was either downward and medially or horizontal, to a downward and lateral inclination (Fig. 4.6). Between 10 and 30° of dorsiflexion, the helical axis ran parallel to a line drawn through the tips of the malleoli, similar to the "empirical axis" of Inman (3). Some subjects had two distinct axes, one for dorsiflexion and one for plantar flexion, whereas in others a more continuous pattern through the whole arc of rotation was seen. The greatest difference in the position of the coronal plane axis between plantar flexion and dorsiflexion ranged between 18 and 63° (mean 37°). Projected onto the horizontal plane, the axis

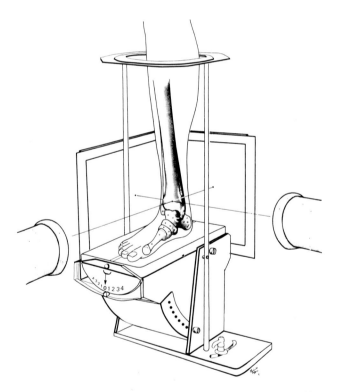

**Figure 4.5.**   Roentgen stereophotogrammetry apparatus with a leg in position and x-ray tubes placed for anteroposterior and lateral exposures against a reference grid. The *dots* in the ankle and foot represent implanted radiopaque marker beads. (From Lundberg et al. The axis of rotation of the ankle joint. J Bone Joint Surg 1989;71-B:95.)

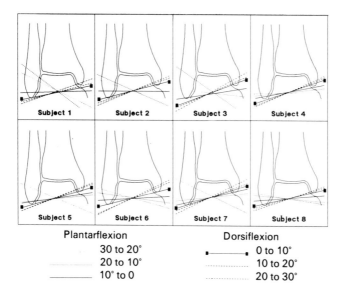

Plantarflexion          Dorsiflexion
  ............  30 to 20°        •——————•  0 to 10°
  ————————  20 to 10°        ...............  10 to 20°
  ————————  10° to 0         .............  20 to 30°

**Figure 4.6.** Individual discrete helical axes of the ankle joint of eight normal subjects for each 10° interval from 30° of plantar flexion to 30° of dorsiflexion, projected onto a coronal plane. (From Lundberg et al. The axis of rotation of the ankle joint. J Bone Joint Surg 1989;71-B:96.)

always ran close to the tips of the malleoli (Fig. 4.7). When projected onto the sagittal plane, differences in inclination between the axes were considerable (6) (Fig. 4.8).

Ankle motion was also measured when the foot was moved from pronation to supination. When projected onto a horizontal plane, the tibio-talar joint axes ran uniformly through the malleoli. In the coronal and sagittal plane, the axes were variable (6).

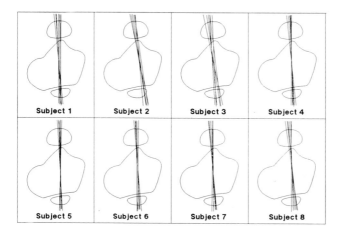

**Figure 4.7.** Individual discrete helical axes projected onto a horizontal plane in eight normal subjects. Axes tend to fall parallel to a transverse plane through the center of the malleoli. (From Lundberg et al. The axis of rotation of the ankle joint. J Bone Joint Surg 1989;71-B:96.)

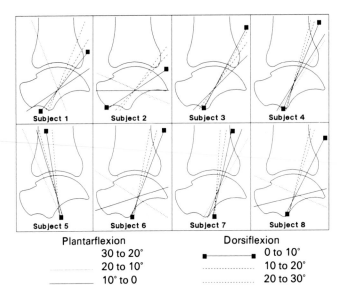

**Figure 4.8.** Individual discrete helical axes projected onto a sagittal plane in eight normal subjects. Variations in inclination are large because axes are viewed almost end-on. (From Lundberg et al. The axis of rotation of the ankle joint. J Bone Joint Surg 1989;71-B:97.)

Ankle motion with medial and lateral rotation of the leg was measured. With lateral rotation of the leg, between 20° of medial rotation and the neutral position, substantial rotation took place at the talo-crural joint. Inclinations of the axes found in medial and lateral rotation, related to the coronal plane, ranged from 1 to 88°, and the range of motion was as much as 16°. Projections of the axes onto the horizontal and sagittal planes were similar to those seen in dorsiflexion and plantar flexion (6).

Probably the most significant finding from the study by Lundberg et al. (6) was that, when plantar flexion and dorsiflexion, pronation and supination, and medial and lateral rotation axes for each subject were drawn in the same figure, all axes, irrespective of their inclination, coincided or ran very close to one central point in the trochlea of the talus (Fig. 4.9). This central point was located at, or slightly lateral to, the midpoint of a line drawn between the tips of the malleoli and seemed to constitute a hub, around which the ankle joint has more freedom of movement than is often assumed.

In a second study, Lundberg et al. (5) studied the kinematics of the ankle/foot complex in the same group of eight volunteers by roentgen stereophotogrammetry in the weight-bearing position. Measurements were made in a three-axis coordinate system (Fig. 4.10) in 10° steps of motion from 30° of plantar flexion to 30° of dorsiflexion. The results are summarized in Table 4.1. From 30° of plantar flexion to the neutral position, dorsiflexion around the transverse axis ranged from 17.5 to 40.1°, with an average of 27.9°. In most subjects, there was a pattern of initial internal rotation around the vertical axis up to 10° of plantar flexion, followed by external rotation from this position to the neutral position (Fig. 4.11). A consistent supinatory rotation around the anteroposterior axis also occurred.

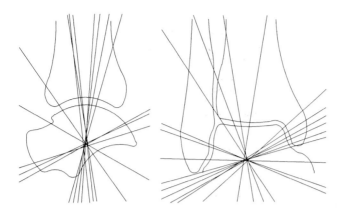

**Figure 4.9.** All coronal and sagittal plane projections of plantar flexion and dorsiflexion, pronation and supination, and medial and lateral rotation axes as seen in a single normal subject. Note the tendency of the axes to cross in one small area within the talus. Similar patterns were observed in most of the other seven subjects. (From Lundberg et al. The axis of rotation of the ankle joint. J Bone Joint Surg 1989;71-B:98.)

From the neutral position to 30° of dorsiflexion (Table 4.1), the resulting rotation around the transverse axis was slightly more than two-thirds of the input rotation (i.e., one-third of the rotation took place at adjacent joints in the foot). There was a consistent pattern of external rotation about the vertical axis but minimal supinatory rotation around the anteroposterior axis.

The axes of rotation of the ankle as defined in a three-plane coordinate system demonstrate a combined motion about all three axes as the foot is moved from plantar

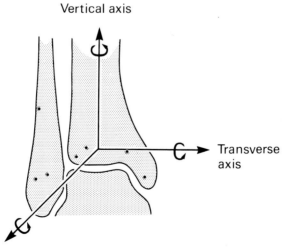

**Figure 4.10.** Three-plane coordinate system. Motion is in relationship to the tibia. Positive rotation: for the transverse axis is plantar flexion; for the vertical axis is internal rotation; and for the anteroposterior axis is supination. (From Lundberg et al. Kinematics of the ankle/foot complex: Plantarflexion and dorsiflexion. Foot Ankle 1989;9(4):196.)

**Table 4.1.**
**Motion around the three tibio-talar axes at 10° degree increments from 30° of plantar flexion to 30° of dorsiflexion for eight normal subjects.**[a,b]

| | Rotation (°) | | |
|---|---|---|---|
| Input Foot Position | Transverse Axis (means ± S.D.) | Vertical Axis (mean ± S.D.) | Anteroposterior Axis (mean ± S.D.) |
| Plantar flexion | | | |
| 30 | 27.9 ± 7.7 | −0.6 ± 3.0 | −4.3 ± 1.9 |
| 20 | 20.8 ± 4.1 | 0.6 ± 2.4 | −3.7 ± 1.6 |
| 10 | 11.1 ± 1.1 | 1.4 ± 0.9 | −2.2 ± 0.9 |
| Dorsiflexion | | | |
| 10 | −5.9 ± 2.3 | −1.8 ± 0.9 | 0.8 ± 0.6 |
| 20 | −15.6 ± 4.0 | −5.6 ± 1.5 | 1.4 ± 1.3 |
| 30 | −22.7 ± 3.0 | −8.9 ± 1.9 | 1.6 ± 2.0 |

[a]From Lundberg et al. Kinematics of the ankle/foot complex: Plantar flexion and dorsiflexion. Foot Ankle 1989;9(4):197.
[b]Values are given as differences compared with the neutral position. Positive difference between values denotes plantar flexion around the transverse axis, internal rotation around the vertical axis, and supination around the anteroposterior axis.

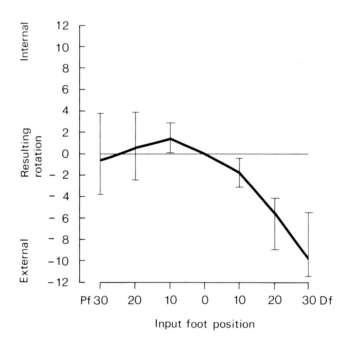

**Figure 4.11.**  Relationship of rotation of the talus around the vertical axis to foot position during ankle dorsiflexion and plantar flexion. Initial pattern of internal rotation followed by marked external rotation. (From Lundberg et al. Kinematics of the ankle/foot complex: Plantarflexion and dorsiflexion. Foot Ankle 9(4):197, 1989.)

flexion to dorsiflexion. The combined motion is complex and shows significant individual variation. However, it is a significant finding that the plantar flexion and dorsiflexion, pronation and supination, and medial and lateral rotation axes for different subjects all seem to fall within one central area in the trochlea of the talus. The existence of this central hub, or center of movement, should have significant implications for placement of the central axis when designing a total ankle prosthesis (6) and for study of the function of the ligaments about the ankle.

## References

1. Barnett CH, Napier JR. The axis of rotation at the ankle joint in man: Its influence upon the form of the talus and the mobility of the fibula. J Anat 1952;86:1.
2. Hicks JH. The mechanics of the foot. I. The joints. J Anat 1953;87:345.
3. Inman VT. The joints of the ankle. Baltimore: Williams & Wilkins, 1976.
4. Isman RE, Inman VT. Anthropometric studies of the human foot and ankle. Biomechanics Laboratory, University of California, San Francisco and Berkeley. Technical Report 58. The Laboratory, San Francisco, 1968.
5. Lundberg A, Goldie I, Kalin B, Selvik G. Kinematics of the ankle/foot complex: Plantarflex-
ion and dorsiflexion. Foot Ankle 1989;9(4):194–200.
6. Lundberg A, Svensson OK, Nemeth G, Selvik G. The axis of rotation of the ankle joint. J Bone Joint Surg 1989;71B:94–99.
7. Sammarco J. Biomechanics of the ankle: Surface velocity and instant center of rotation in the sagittal plane. Am J Sports Med 1977;5(6):231–234.
8. Siegler S, Chen J, Schneck CD. The three dimensional kinematics and flexibility characteristics of the human ankle and subtalar joints. Part I: Kinematics. J Biomech Eng 1988;110:364–373.

# 5

# Subtalar Joint: Morphology and Functional Anatomy

## BRUCE J. SANGEORZAN, M.D.

The subtalar joint is variously called the subtalar, talocalcaneal, or lesser ankle joint. Each name implies a role of this articulation—the first implies its major responsibility in integrating all functions distal to the ankle; the second implies a relatively local importance in articulation of the two tarsal bones of the hindfoot; and the third recognizes that its function is highly integrated with that of the ankle in melding the function of the foot with that of the long bones. The inclusion of a section on the subtalar joint in a text on the ankle is a tribute to its historical role as the "lesser ankle" and a reminder of our relatively unsophisticated understanding of the function of the hindfoot. The subtalar joint does not act alone. In addition to its action in concert with the tibiotalar joint, its motion is integrated with that of the transverse tarsal joint. The latter very complex and important function is not addressed in this work.

## ANATOMY

The anatomy of the subtalar joint, described in depth by Sarrafian (15), includes the talus and calcaneus and their associated soft tissue structures. The talus, which consists of a head, neck, and body, is covered by articular cartilage on 60% of its surface. No extrinsic or intrinsic muscle inserts on the talus. As a result, its kinematics are determined by forces acting across the ankle, talocalcaneal, and talonavicular joints. The subtalar joint consists of three articular facets on the inferior aspect of the talus and superior aspect of the calcaneus. The largest of the three facets is the posterior facet, which, according to Inman, is oriented approximately 37° (range 26–50°) from the transverse axis directed from anterolateral to posteromedial. It forms a saddle-like joint on the underside of the talar body with its concave shape in the long axis and a slightly convex contour in the short axis. Most commonly, this facet is separate from the anterior and middle facet, whereas the latter two are often continuous. There is considerable variation in size and shape of the facets, and all three may be continuous, obliterating the tarsal canal. The anterior and middle facets occupy a position on the underside of the talar neck. The neck generally is 17 mm in length (range

12–23 mm) and is angulated 24° (10–44°) medial to the long axis of the foot, and 24° (5–50°) plantar to a line parallel to the walking surface. There is substantial variation in orientation of the axis of the body versus that of the neck of the talus. These variations may influence the axis and range of motion of the subtalar joint.

The calcaneus has three facets mirroring those of the talus. The middle third of the calcaneus supports the posterior facet. This facet is angulated anteriorly an average of 65°, but Inman noted "remarkable variation" in the orientation. In particular, he noted that only 58% exhibited the oblique helicoid or "screw-shaped" surface described by Manter (10). (This shape, which causes forward translation with rotatory movements, is discussed in the motion section of this chapter.) The anterior third of the calcaneus is covered by the anterior and middle articular facets. These support the underside of the talar neck and head and have not been as well described.

In addition to bony anatomy, function of the subtalar joint is influenced by the extensive ligament and soft tissue support within and around the subtalar joint. The important soft tissues include the joint capsule, interosseus talocalcaneal ligament, the lateral, medial, and posterior talocalcaneal ligaments, the flexor and extensor retinacula, the extrinsic tendons that cross the subtalar joint, as well as ligaments bridging the transverse tarsal joint. Some of the ligaments that bind the talus to the calcaneus, such as the deltoid ligament, function as part of the overall talocalcaneal-navicular complex. This bony triumvirate functions as a unit in the mechanics of the

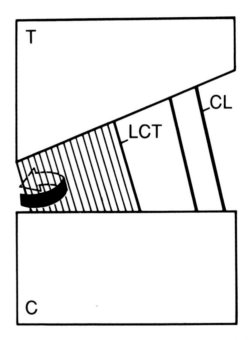

**Figure 5.1.**   A thematic representation of the talocalcaneal ligament (*TCL*) and cervical ligament (*CL*). The short medial fibers act as a pivot point as the talus rotates on the calcaneus. The outer fibers, including the cervical ligament have a greater excursion. *T*, talus; *C*, calcaneus. (From Sarrafian SK. Anatomy of the foot and ankle. Philadelphia: JB Lippincott, 1983.)

hindfoot. However, a discussion of the transverse tarsal joint is beyond the depth of discussion of this chapter.

The interosseus talocalcaneal ligament, also known as the ligament of the tarsal canal, is a flat, oblique band that originates in the tarsal canal close to the anterior capsule of the posterior facet. The fibers are directed obliquely upward and medially, and insert into the sulcus of the talus. The interosseous talocalcaneal ligament is joined by a lateral and a posterior talocalcaneal ligament and by the stout cervical ligament in providing stability without completely obliterating translation and rotation. These ligaments average 15–20 mm in length and are generally oriented in a similar oblique fashion. The ligament of the tarsal canal is shorter than the more externally positioned cervical ligament. The combination of the oblique orientation and relative lengths of the ligaments allows the talus to pivot around the short medial ligaments until the cervical ligament comes under tension. The fibers' oblique orientation becomes more vertical when the hindfoot is inverted (Fig. 5.1), which places the cervical ligament under tension. As a result, when in this position, relatively little rotatory motion can occur between the bones.

## Motion at the Subtalar Joint

In the previous edition of this book, Inman stated, "Considerable confusion seems to persist as to the type of movement that occurs between the talus and calcaneus." He identified three roadblocks to clarification of the motion: the motion occurs outside the usual planes of joint motion, the language used to describe the motion is ambiguous, and the actual understanding of the motion is limited. Unfortunately, very little information has been added to the literature to clarify the confusion since then.

Talocalcaneal motion can be divided into angular, linear, and rotational parts (7). Since there was such substantial variation in the terms used to describe the motion, it is impossible to have a clear understanding of the older literature. But it appears that some authors felt that rotation was not possible. Frazer (5) implied that no rotation was possible due to the orientation of the articular surfaces and only a forward and inward gliding of the talus on the calcaneus took place. He also stated that no rocking and no side-to-side motion was possible. Gray (6) agreed that the motion was limited to sliding but thought the bones could slide side to side as well.

Quain (13), Peirsol (12), and Cunningham (1) agreed that the primary motion of the subtalar joint was a rotation about an oblique axis that centered in the area of the interosseus ligament but disagreed about the direction of the axis. Hollinshead (8) reiterated this information and cited its importance in allowing inversion and eversion of the posterior part of the foot. Inman credits Meyer (11), in his writings in German, with the first clear description of the axis of rotation, including its position as projected in the sagittal and transverse planes.

These concepts were first introduced in the English language literature by Elftman and Manter (2) in a treatise on the anatomy and function of the foot. A more precise definition of the axis of the subtalar joint was achieved by Manter (10) using available technology and largely visual measurements of instrumented cadaver specimens. In his 16 specimens, he noted the inclination of the axis of the subtalar joint to be 42° (range 29–47°) as measured upward from the horizontal plane and projected on the sagittal plane, and deviating 16° (range 8–24°) medially from a line connecting the midpoint of the heel to the first web space, then projected onto the transverse plane. But even among his 16 specimens he found considerable variation.

Isman and Inman (9), using a similar technique, measured 46 cadaver feet. (They later extended their study to include more than 100 feet without any significant change.) Their average angles were very similar—42° vertical and 23° medial—with a slightly larger medial deviation being accounted for by their use of the midline of the foot rather than the first web space as a landmark (Figs. 5.2 and 5.3). These authors also noted substantial individual variation. In their series, range of measurements was 20–68° in the sagittal plane and 4–47° of medial deviation (transverse plane). Inman summarized this information by stating that "it now appears well-established that motion between the talus and the calcaneus is a rotatory one about a single oblique axis." Motion that occurs about this oblique axis is associated with one of two groups: pronation, abduction, extension; or supination, adduction, and flexion.

Somewhat more controversial is the question of screw-like motion of the subtalar joint. This means that the rotation of the talus on the calcaneus is accompanied by anterior and posterior translation, just as a screw moves forward as it is turned (Fig.

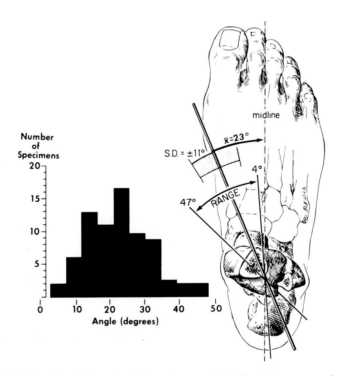

**Figure 5.2.** Variations in position of subtalar axis as projected onto transverse plane. The angle was measured between the axis and the midline of the foot. The extent of individual variation is shown on the sketch and revealed in the histogram.

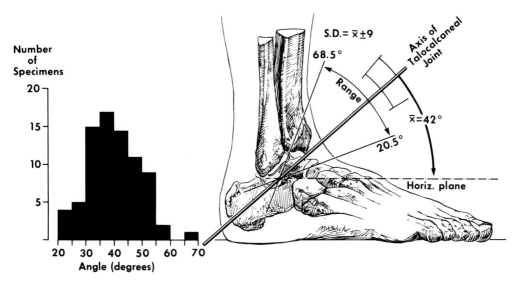

**Figure 5.3.** Variations in inclination of axis of subtalar joint as projected upon sagittal plane. The distribution of the measurements on the individual specimens is shown in the histogram. The single observation of an angle of almost 70° was present in a markedly cavus foot.

5.4). Manter summarized the principles involved as follows. If the congruity of two surfaces is to be maintained with movement, and movement is in a plane oblique to the joint axis, the motion must include a lateral translation or screw-like rotation (4). Since the articular orientation and ligament constraint of the talocalcaneal joint doesn't allow lateral translation, Manter felt screw-like motion must occur. As evidence for this motion, he noted that serial sections of the posterior facet of the calcaneus made perpendicular to the joint axis formed spiral rather than circular arcs. And, he noted that the anterior and middle facets form a shallow trough that allowed the talar neck to slide and rotate. Based on these anatomic findings, his measurements of the relative lengths of the bones and their total rotation, he calculated that the anterior displacement of the talus occurring in pronation approximated 1.5 mm for each 10° of rotation in the joint (10). The shape of the posterior facet and its congruity with the talar surface are critical to this motion. If the posterior facet acts as a screw, it should show constant increments of longitudinal displacement with continuing rotation. The later assumption is apparently not true (16). The posterior facet is congruous in a neutral position but is incongruous at the limits of its motion. Inman believed that the incongruence was not enough to affect the validity of the hypothesis and attempted to validate the screw-like motion by studies of the facet anatomy using a larger number of specimens. He contoured the articular surface of cadaver specimens and plotted the linear displacement versus their degrees of rotation. Approximately 58% of his specimens exhibited some incremental anterior forward motion of the talus with pronation, 20% initially exhibited negative translation followed by positive, another 20% showed a back and forth type motion, whereas 3% exhibited pure rotatory motion. More recent studies in our laboratory have demonstrated the large variation

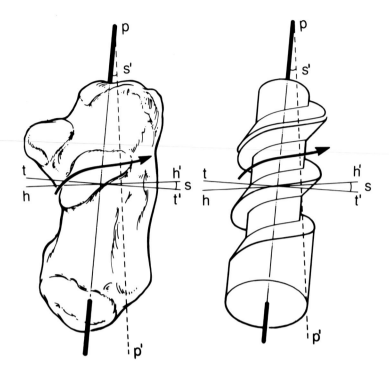

**Figure 5.4.** Comparison of a right posterior facet with a right-handed screw. As the screw is turned in a clockwise direction, it advances. *hh'* is the horizontal plane in which motion is occurring. *tt'* is a plane perpendicular to the axis of the screw. *s* is the helix angle of the screw formed by the intersection of *hh'* and *tt'* and is equal to *s'*, which is obtained by dropping a perpendicular *pp'* from the axis. (From Manter JT. Movements of the subtalar and transverse tarsal joints. Anat Rec 1941;80:397−410.

in the motion of the talocalcaneal joint while under load. To further cloud the issue, the axis of motion varies within the same specimen when the direction of load is changed.

By direct measurement of talar excursion on a fixed calcaneus independent of facet orientation, Inman found that only one in five specimens exhibited continuous incremental anterior motion and could therefore be described as screw-like. This difference between predicted and measured translation indicated that the motion reflects both the shape of the calcaneus and that of the talus. Of the 20% of specimens that did exhibit the continuous displacement, the average pitch was about 2/3 of that calculated by Manter and 1/2 the value that would have been calculated from the contour of the calcaneus alone.

In vivo, there is no discrete separation between the motion of the talocalcaneal joint and that of the tibiotalar articulation. The range of motion of the foot shank complex in any direction is greater than that of either the ankle or subtalar joint alone (3). This is due to kinematic coupling. Siegler et al. (14) conducted studies on 15 fresh amputation lower limbs. They found that neither the ankle or subtalar joint acts with a fixed axis of rotation. Motion of the foot shank complex in any direction occurs by combined motion of both joints. They strongly stated that a single fixed axis of rotation is an inappropriate method to describe subtalar joint motion. The authors collected data on a fresh cadaver foot fixed into a testing apparatus with a fixed tibial reference frame using a position data acquisition system with a three-dimensional sonic digitizer, combined with a system of six pneumatic actuators. The authors found that the subtalar joint contributed about 20% of the motion of the hindfoot to dorsiflexion-plantar flexion, and that this contribution occurred primarily at the extremes of the range of motion. In inversion and eversion, the majority of the motion occurs through the subtalar joint, but at extremes the ankle joint contributes. However, the contribution of the subtalar joint is approximately equal to that of the ankle joint in internal and external rotation. This study did not fix the foot in a neutral position, and the joints were under no load at the time of testing.

## RANGE OF MOTION AT THE SUBTALAR JOINT

Difficulties arise in measuring the motion of the subtalar joint from (*a*) variation in subtalar axis and anatomy, (*b*) coupling with the ankle joint, and (*c*) definition of neutral position. In testing living subjects, direct measurement cannot be done without fixing instruments to bone. The size of the bone coupled with its limited motion make the measurement error from the mobile soft tissue interface relatively important. When instrumented cadaver specimens are used to enhance accuracy, the outcome is influenced by embalming and preservation methods and occult pathology. Both methods are influenced by the variations in the subtalar joint axis. If the hinge of the measurement device, i.e., goniometer, is not aligned with center of motion of the joint, the measurement device will restrict motion. As a result, there is substantial variation in measured range of motion.

In a study of 102 cadaver specimens, Inman found the range of motion varied from 10 to 59° with an average of 24 ± 11°. In 50 living subjects (100 ankles) the range averaged 40 + 7° (range 20–65°). The latter measurement was made with a goniometer attached to the hindfoot and could not distinguish between the ankle and subtalar joint. The large difference could be attributed to stiffness induced by preservation methods in the cadaver study or to kinematic coupling with the ankle joint in the study of living subjects. Inman chose to stress the wide variability of motion in the subtalar joint. He cautioned the examiner to remember that when evaluating an individual patient, 10–60° of motion could be considered normal. Comparison to the individual's other foot can be helpful.

### References

1. Cunningham DJ. Cunningham's Text-Book of Anatomy. 5th ed. Robinson A, ed. New York: William Wood and Co., 1927.
2. Elftman H, Manter J. The evolution of the human foot, with especial reference to the joints. J Anat 1935;70:56.
3. Engsberg JR. A biomechanical analysis of the talocalcaneal joint – In vitro. J Biomech 1987;20:429–442.
4. Fick R. Handbuch der Anatomie und Mechanik der Gelenke unter Berücksichtigung der bewegenden Muskeln, Part 1. Jena: Gustav Fischer Verlag, 1904.
5. Frazer JE. The anatomy of the human skeleton. London: J. & A. Churchill, 1965.
6. Gray H. Anatomy of the Human Body. 29th ed. Goss CM, ed. Philadelphia: Lea & Febiger, 1973.

7. Hicks JH. The mechanics of the foot. I. The joints. J Anat 1953;87:345.

8. Hollinshead WH. Textbook of Anatomy. 2nd ed. New York: Harper & Row, 1967.

9. Isman RE, Inman VT. Anthropometric studies of the human foot and ankle. Biomechanics Laboratory, University of California, San Francisco and Berkeley. Technical Report 58. The Laboratory, San Francisco, 1968.

10. Manter, JT. Movements of the subtalar and transverse tarsal joints. Anat Rec 1941;80:397.

11. Meyer H. Das aufrechte Gehen (Zweiter Beitrag zur Mechanik des menschlichen Knochengerüstes). Arch Anat Physiol Wissensch. Med 1853; p. 365.

12. Piersol GA. Human anatomy, including structure and development and practical considerations. 8th ed. Philadelphia: JB Lippincott, 1923.

13. Quain's elements of anatomy. 10th ed. vol. 2, part 2. Schäfer EA, Thane GD, eds. London: Longmans, Green & Co., 1892.

14. Siegler S, Chen J, Schenck CD. The three dimensional kinematics and flexibility characteristics of the human ankle and subtalar joint. Part I: Kinematics. J Biomech Eng 1988;110:364–373.

15. Sarrafian SK. Anatomy of the foot and ankle. Philadelphia: JB Lippincott, 1983.

16. Huson A. Een ontleedkundig-functioneel onderzoek van de voetwortel: An anatomical and functional study of the tarsal joints. Leiden: Luctor et Emergo, 1961.

# 6

# Biomechanics of the Ankle Joint

## JAMES B. STIEHL, M.D.

### SIMPLE KINEMATICS OF THE ANKLE JOINT

To describe the basic kinematic relationships that exists in the ankle joint, Inman utilized a simple model consisting of a hinge joint with a single axis. The leg was represented by a vertical wooden member and the foot was constructed as a single wooden piece shaped to resemble the shape of the foot. It is understood that such a simplistic presentation of the ankle does not accurately reproduce the true anatomic conditions that exist in any single individual, but by selecting the extremes of variability from his anthropometric studies, the effects of various positions are exaggerated.

From the model, we see that the midline of the foot is indicated by a black line on its dorsal and plantar surfaces. The hinge connects the lower leg to the foot, and a calibrated disc is attached to the bottom of the foot. By varying the position of the hinge joint in the coronal and transverse planes, we can understand the effects of anatomical difference (Fig. 6.1). From Chapter 4, we know that the axis of the ankle joint does not remain a fixed point as would be defined by a simple hinge, but the practical representation of the ankle mechanics in motion is accurate. In the following series of pictures, the foot is either free to move in directions dictated by the hinge or is fixed to the ground and immobile while the lower leg moves upon the foot.

### Foot Free, Leg Fixed

**Variable Position of Ankle Axis in Relation to Fixed Knee Axis.** The axis of the knee joint has been utilized to represent a fixed plane to measure the variabilities of the ankle joint as projected onto the transverse plane. In adults, the average inclination of the ankle joint in relation to the knee joint is approximately 23° of "external tibial torsion" where the ankle joint axis is inclined laterally and posteriorly. Individual angular differences are great and may vary as much as 30° on either side of the mean. The basic model has a pivot joint located just above the ankle hinge joint to simulate a typical amount of tibial "internal" or "external" torsion. In this situation, the leg is fixed, and the foot is rotated 25° to represent this effect of torsion. We can observe the effect of plantar and dorsiflexion of the ankle by watching the transparent plastic disc. A "Devil Level" is fixed to the foot aligned at a right angle to the midline of the foot to demonstrate any rotatory displacements. The three views

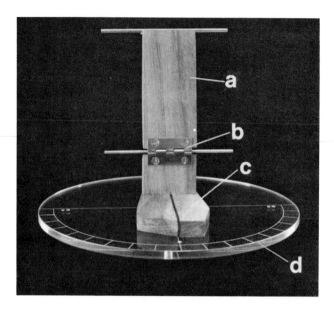

**Figure 6.1.** Photograph of basic model to be used in demonstrating effects of variations in position of ankle axis. The vertical wooden member (*a*) represents the leg. It carries on its upper end a short metal rod that represents the axis of the knee joint. The hinge (*b*) represents the ankle joint. The pin of the hinge has been extended for easier reference. The foot (*c*) is represented by a horizontal wooden member roughly shaped to resemble a right foot and is attached to the ankle hinge by a short vertical piece. The midline of the foot is shown as a black line. Fixed to the foot is a plastic disk (*d*) calibrated in 10° increments from the zero position, which is the sagittal plane of the foot and leg. The inscribed diameter of the disk that connects the two 90° calibrations will always be kept in the same vertical plane as the knee axis. The amount of toeing in or toeing out can be determined by noting the position of the black line on the foot in relation to the calibrations on the disk.

shown demonstrate neutral, 20° of dorsiflexion, and 30° of plantar flexion. From the models, we see that, if the axis of the hinge remains horizontal and in a fixed position of 90° to the midline of the foot, there is no rotation of the foot about its long axis with dorsiflexion or plantar flexion. The foot is simply toed in or toed out in relation to the fixed knee axis (Figs. 6.2 and 6.3).

**Variable Position of Ankle Axis in Relation to Midline of the Foot.** Most anatomy textbooks state that the ankle axis is directed posterolateral in relation to the midline of the foot in the horizontal plane. Inman's anthropometric studies on cadaver specimens found that the average posterolateral deviation of the ankle axis from the midline of the foot was 6°. Individual variation is considerable and posterolateral inclination as great as 20° was seen, whereas in a few specimens the inclination was reversed anterolaterally a few degrees. We can see the effect of changing the relationship of the ankle joint axis and the midline of the foot by observing photographs of the model. In these examples, the knee joint and ankle joint axis are fixed in parallel position. Only the foot is rotated medially or laterally in relation to the

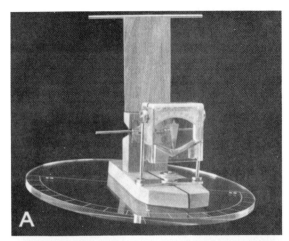

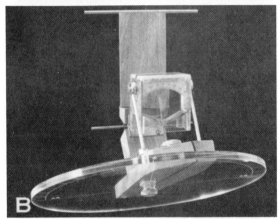

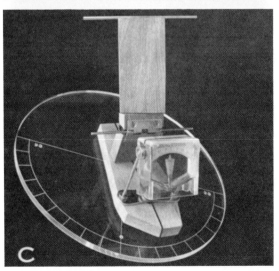

**Figure 6.2.** Series of photographs of model in Figure 6.1 showing ankle hinge with its attached foot rotated medially 25° in relation to knee axis. The diameter inscribed on the plastic disk, connecting the 90° marks, remains in the plane of the knee axis. The medial rotation of the foot of 25° is readily seen by relating the position of the black line on the foot to the inscribed 10° increments on the pastic disk. The ankle hinge is at a right angle to the midline of the foot and the Devil Level remains parallel to the ankle hinge. The vertical plane of motion dictated by the ankle hinge is now no longer in the sagittal plane of the leg but in a new vertical plane rotated medially 25° from the knee axis. From the neutral position (**A**), the model is dorsiflexed 20° (**B**), and plantar flexed 30° (**C**). The following particulars should be noted. The plane of movement is now oblique to the coronal plane as determined by the knee axis. The plane of movement as depicted by the plastic disk and projected onto the coronal plane appears to tilt on dorsiflexion and plantar flexion of the foot. However, the Devil Level, which remains parallel to the ankle axis, reveals that no rotation of the foot about its long axis occurs.

**Figure 6.3.** Effect of rotating foot of model laterally 25° in relation to knee axis. Again note that dorsiflexion (**B**) and plantar flexion (**C**) of the foot occur in a vertical plane that is oblique to the sagittal plane of the leg. The inclinations of the plastic disk are reversed from those in Figure 6.2, but there is still no rotation of the foot about its long axis as revealed by the Devil Level. The foot is simply dorsiflexing and plantar flexing in a plane that is oblique to the sagittal plane of the leg.

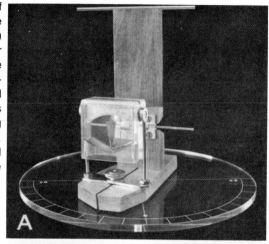

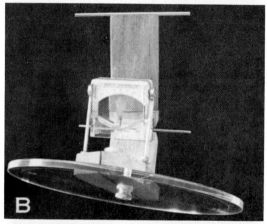

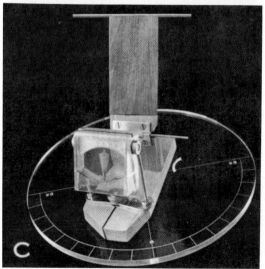

ankle hinge (Figs. 6.4 and 6.5). From study of the photographs, we note that deviations of the midline of the foot from the neutral axis of the ankle joint cause rotation of the foot about its long axis. The amount of rotation of the foot varies as the sine of the angle of deviation of the foot from the sagittal plane of the leg.

**Variable Position of the Ankle Axis in the Coronal Plane.** The axis of the ankle joint is rarely ever horizontal when projected onto the coronal plane. It is inclined downward from the medial to the lateral side. The degree of obliquity has an average inclination of 12° with a maximum inclination of 23°. In the model, the hinge is oriented downward and laterally at a 23° angle to demonstrate the greatest contrast, and the knee axis and the midline of the foot remain parallel to the hinge (Fig. 6.6). With dorsiflexion and plantar flexion, we note essentially no longitudinal rotation of the foot. However, there is toe out of the foot with dorsiflexion and toe in with plantar flexion. In the next model, the plastic disk and Devil Level have been removed and the dorsiflexion and plantar flexion increased to 40°. The foot toeing in and toeing out become obvious (Fig. 6.7).

**Effect of Combining Axial Positions in Transverse and Coronal Planes.** In the normal living person, the ankle axis is obliquely oriented in both the transverse and coronal planes when related to the foot. We then combine the last two examples and find that the ankle axis is inclined downward from the medial to lateral side and backward in relation to the midline of the foot. Inman investigated individual angular values from 46 cadaver feet and found no correlation between the obliquity of the ankle axis in the coronal plane and the amount of the deviation of the midline of the foot in the transverse plane. Thus, they function as independent variables and can be separated as we have seen in the above examples. Deviation of the midline of the foot from the neutral right angle of the ankle axis causes longitudinal rotation of the foot with dorsiflexion and plantar flexion (pronation and supination). Similarly, change of the axis of the ankle in the coronal plane causes the foot to toe out in dorsiflexion and toe in on plantar flexion (Figs. 6.8 and 6.9).

### Foot Fixed, Leg Free

**Effect of an Oblique Axis of the Ankle upon the Leg with the Foot Fixed.** During the stance phase of walking, the effect of the oblique ankle axis is on the lower leg rather than the foot. The following examples demonstrate the net effect of simple plantar flexion and dorsiflexion of the foot with the various orientations of the ankle axis. The final demonstration will show the rotatory displacement of the lower leg that occurs with stance phase dorsiflexion and plantar flexion.

**Effect of Varying the Axis in the Transverse Plane.** If the ankle axis were placed in a horizontal plane parallel to the axis of the knee and at a right angle to the midline of the foot, we observe that the entire range of motion of the leg occurs directly in the sagittal plane. No rotation of the leg about the vertical will occur (Fig. 6.10). If the axis of the ankle rotates medially or laterally in relation to the fixed foot, the new plane of movement will deviate either medially or laterally from the sagittal plane. The net effect is to cause the leg to incline laterally from the sagittal plane on dorsiflexion and medially from the sagittal on plantar flexion (Fig. 6.11).

**Effect of an Oblique Axis in Both the Sagittal and Coronal Plane.** Anthropometric studies have demonstrated that the normal axis of the ankle always

**Figure 6.4.** Ankle (hinge) and knee axes parallel and in same vertical (coronal) plane. The foot has been rotated medially 25° to the coronal plane of the ankle hinge. Attention is directed to the Devil Level, which shows that in dorsiflexion (**B**) and plantar flexion (**C**) there is rotation of the foot about its long axis. The direction of this rotation on dorsiflexion is a pronatory one. The longitudinal rotation in plantar flexion is in a reverse direction (supinatory).

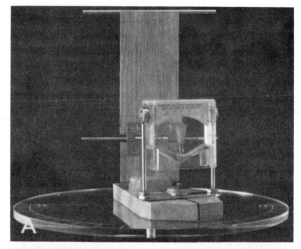

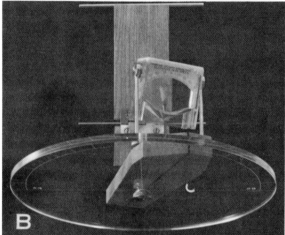

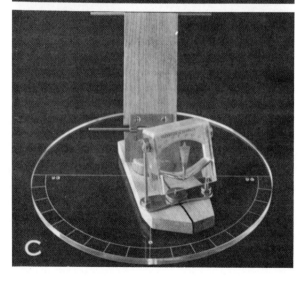

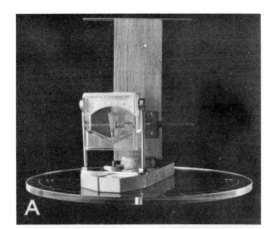

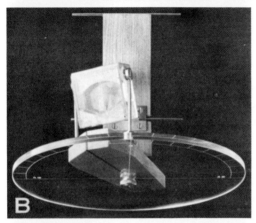

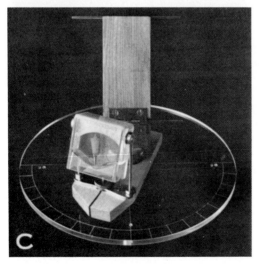

**Figure 6.5.** Same projections of model as in Figure 6.4. The foot, however, has been rotated laterally in relation to the ankle axis by 25°. Reference to the Devil Level demonstrates that again there is a rotation of the foot about its long axis on dorsiflexion and plantar flexion. The direction of this rotation is opposite to that shown in Figure 6.4.

**Figure 6.6.** Modification of wooden model by replacement of horizontal hinge with hinge that is inclined 23° to horizontal. The knee axis and the ankle hinge remain in the same vertical plane. The midline of the foot is at a right angle to this plane. Attention is directed to the Devil Level. Note that on dorsiflexion and on plantar flexion there is little longitudinal rotation of the foot about its long axis. The foot toes slightly outward on dorsiflexion (**B**) and slightly inward on plantar flexion (**C**).

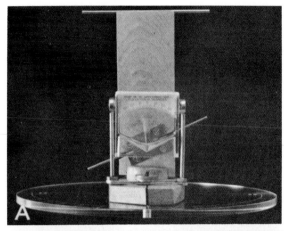

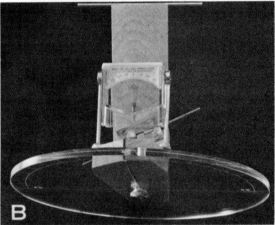

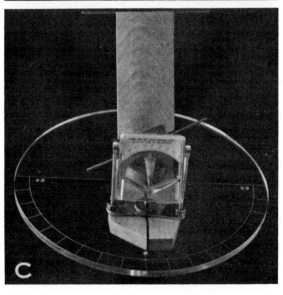

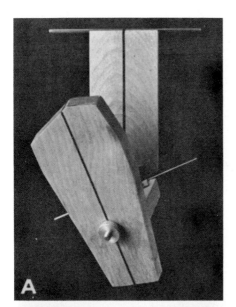

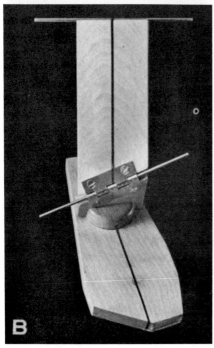

**Figure 6.7.** Same arrangement of model as in Figure 6.6. For the sake of clarity, the plastic disk and Devil Level have been removed and a black line has been inscribed on the vertical member to indicate the midline of the leg. Dorsiflexion to 40° is shown in **A** and plantar flexion to 40° in **B**. The toeing out on dorsiflexion and toeing in on plantar flexion, which result from the obliquity of the hinge, are clearly shown.

**Figure 6.8.** Foot rotated medially 25°
in relation to oblique axis of ankle hinge.
During dorsiflexion and plantar flexion
of the ankle, the vertical displacement
of the foot will occur in a plane oblique
by 25° to the plane of the ankle hinge.
It will be seen that dorsiflexion and
plantar flexion impose a longitudinal rotation of the foot as revealed by the
Devil Level. Note that this longitudinal
rotation is similar to that shown in Figure 6.4 and is due to the 25° of medial
rotation of the foot. To this longitudinal
rotation of the foot is added the toeing-
in effect of the obliquely oriented ankle
hinge (see Figs. 6.6 and 6.7); this is
emphasized in Figure 6.7.

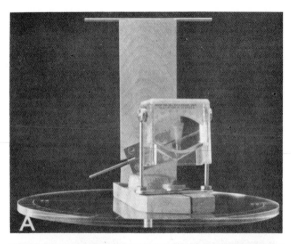

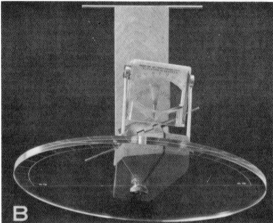

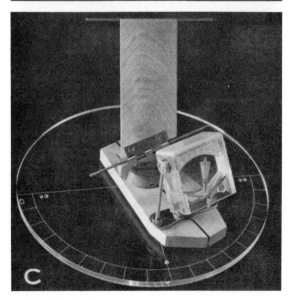

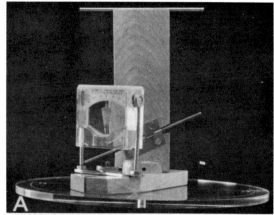

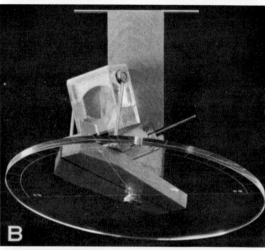

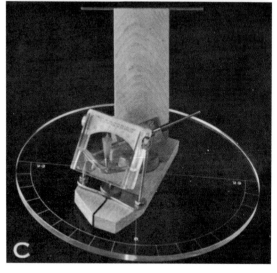

**Figure 6.9.** Foot rotated laterally 25° in relation to axis of ankle joint. This orientation has caused a longitudinal rotation of the foot about its long axis, but in a reverse direction. Note that there is still a tendency for the foot to rotate medially during plantar flexion because of flexion about the obliquely oriented hinge.

**Figure 6.10.** Wooden model seen from above. The foot is fixed and the leg is moved from a neutral position (**A**) to dorsiflexion of 20° (**B**) and to plantar flexion of 30° (**C**). Note that the pins indicating the knee and ankle axes remain parallel. Movement occurs in the sagittal plane. There is no rotation of the leg about its vertical axis.

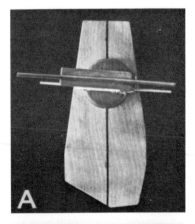

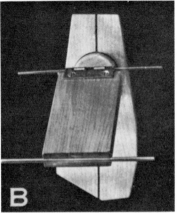

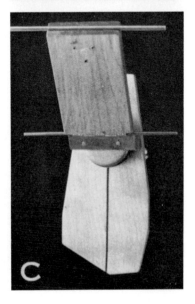

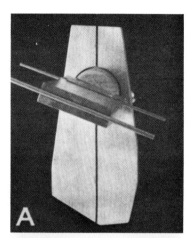

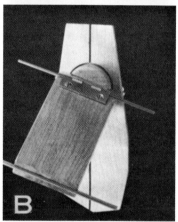

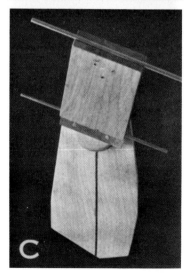

**Figure 6.11.** Model with axes of knee and ankle laterally rotated in relation to midline of foot. Note that the leg again shows no rotation about a vertical axis. This is evident from the parallelism that persists between the pins that locate the knee and ankle axes. The leg moves in a plane that is oblique to the sagittal plane. This causes the leg to deviate laterally on dorsiflexion (**B**) and medially on plantar flexion (**C**).

**Figure 6.12.** Ankle hinge oriented obliquely in coronal plane. The orientation is the same as in Figures 6.6–6.9. The pins representing the knee and ankle axes are at a right angle to the midline of the foot. The effect of the oblique hinge causes a rotation of the leg about a vertical axis during movement of the leg over the fixed foot. From the neutral position (**A**), where the axes of the knee and ankle are parallel, note that on dorsiflexion (**B**) the leg rotates medially relative to the foot. On plantar flexion (**C**) the leg rotates laterally relative to the foot.

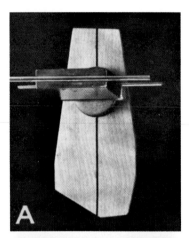

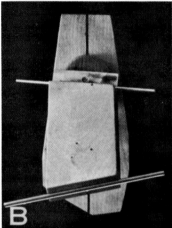

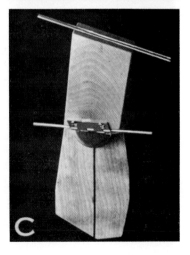

inclines laterally and downward from medial to lateral in the coronal plane. With the foot fixed in stance phase, dorsiflexion at the ankle causes medial rotation of the lower leg, and plantar flexion causes lateral rotation of the lower leg. We see very little tendency for inclination of the lower leg out of the sagittal plane as seen from the last example. Thus, the anatomical orientation of the ankle joint axis allows the lower leg to pass through space, remaining very close to the sagittal plane with range of motion over the fixed foot (Fig. 6.12). However, there is significant rotation of the lower leg to allow this to occur. The following anatomical specimen clearly demonstrates this phenomenon. We can see that the anteroposterior inserted pins diverge or demonstrate external rotation of the lower leg with plantar flexion and converge showing internal rotation of the lower leg with dorsiflexion (Figs. 6.13 and 6.14).

## Clinical Application to Human Locomotion

To understand the complexity of the oblique ankle joint axis is to realize that mere dorsiflexion or plantar flexion in the sagittal plane is a gross oversimplification. We can observe from the above models that complex rotatory displacements occur in the leg and foot with ambulation. The stance phase of normal walking clearly demonstrates some of these motions. The stance phase can be divided into three intervals. The first interval occurs from heel strike to foot flat. The second interval is from foot flat to the instant of heel rise. The third interval is from the beginning of heel rise to toe-off.

**First Interval.** At the time of heel strike, the entire lower extremity rotates medially and the foot plantar flexes from a position of slight dorsiflexion. Until the foot is immobilized by friction with the floor, it is free to move in space and, depending on the obliquity of the ankle joint, will tend to toe in to a varying degree.

**Second Interval.** The foot is flat on the floor, and as the leg passes over the weight-bearing foot, there is dorsiflexion in the ankle joint. From the above model,

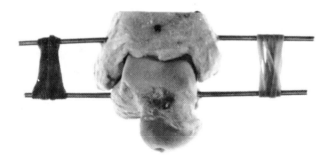

**Figure 6.13.** Anatomic preparation demonstrating that an oblique axis of ankle joint causes horizontal rotation about a vertical axis between talus and leg when ankle is dorsiflexed and plantar flexed. A randomly selected specimen was used. The tibia and fibula have been cut just proximal to the ankle mortise and articulated within the talus. The articular surfaces of the ankle are held in firm apposition with rubber bands as shown in the photograph. The talus was securely fixed by a 6.4-mm bolt passed through its neck and attached to a metal base, leaving the tibia and fibula free to move.

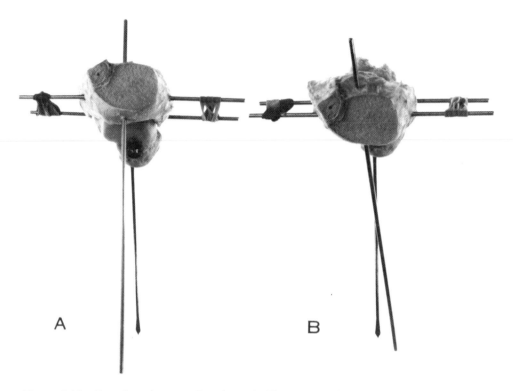

**Figure 6.14.**  Top view of preparation shown in Figure 10.13. Metal rods have been inserted into the talar head and the tibia to act as pointers. In **A**, the ankle is in plantar flexion. Note that the two points diverge. In **B**, the ankle is in full dorsiflexion. Note that horizontal rotation of the tibia on the talus has occurred, with crossing of the pointers.

we can see that with dorsiflexion of the ankle joint with the foot fixed there is medial rotation of the leg about a vertical axis.

**Third Interval.**  As the heel rises, the motion of the ankle joint is relative plantar flexion. Again from the above model of the fixed foot, we see that this motion causes the leg to rotate laterally. This lateral rotation of the leg occurs until toe-off.

In summary, the oblique ankle axis produces toe in from plantar flexion that occurs from the instant of heel contact to the time the foot is flat. During midstance, relative dorsiflexion of the ankle joint occurs as the foot is fixed to the ground. Medial rotation of the leg occurs as the leg passes over the foot. As the heel rises, plantar flexion occurs, which results in lateral rotation of the leg on a fixed foot (Fig. 6.15).

In normal locomotion, ankle motion ranges from 20 to 36°, with an average of 24°. The obliquity of the ankle axis ranges from 2 to 23°, with an average of 12° from the horizontal. With the most oblique ankle joint axis and the maximum range of movement possible, only about 11° of rotation of the leg occurs about the vertical axis. Independent observations of normal lower leg rotation in walking demonstrate considerably higher values than can be explained from the oblique axis of the ankle alone even in the most exaggerated case. Obviously, the articulations of the subtalar

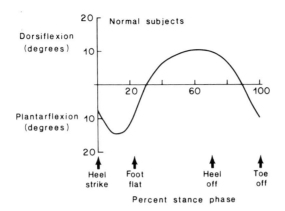

**Figure 6.15.** Mean pattern of ankle joint motion in normal subjects. (From Stauffer R, Chao E, Brewster R. Force and motion analysis of the normal, diseased, and prosthetic ankle joint. Clin Orthop Relat Res 1977;127:193.)

joint and forefoot to a lesser degree play a significant role in horizontal rotation of the lower leg and will be discussed in the next chapter.

## KINETIC ANALYSIS OF THE ANKLE JOINT

From previous work by Frankel and Nordin (3), free body equations have defined the joint reaction forces acting on the ankle joint to be quite high. For example, the joint reaction force resulting from rising up on the tiptoe is about 2.1 times body weight (Fig. 6.16). Stauffer et al. (19) used a two-dimensional "quasi-static" force analysis to calculate joint reaction force in various places of gait (Fig. 6.17). From heel strike to flat foot, the compressive forces rose to about three times body weight. At the period of heel off when pull of the Achilles tendon produced a large plantar flexion movement, calculated values of articular compressive force reached 4.5 to 5.5 (mean 4.73) times body weight. Increasing the stride cadence did not significantly alter this magnitude (Fig. 6.18). Tangential "fore and aft" or shear forces were also documented in the normal gait cycle reaching mean peak value of 36% body weight during the latter phase of foot push off to heel off (19). Procter and Paul (12) used a three-dimensional analysis and found peak resultant forces of 2.91 to 4.67 (mean 3.88) times body weight. The problem with any of these techniques relates to the fact that actual determination of internal forces across the joint surfaces are only estimations.

Weiss et al. (23, 24) investigated the effect of passive dorsiflexion and plantar flexion on the torque resistance generated by these maneuvers in human volunteers. Expectedly, ankle joint stiffness and passive torque generated increased at the extremes of motion while little if any resistance occurred at the neutral midrange points at about 15° of plantar flexion. When active muscle contractions where added to this model, it was found that the actual angle of flexion had little effect on the torque generated. Thus, the active torque resistance and elastic stiffness of the ankle joint remained constant over the entire range of motion. There was, however, a difference

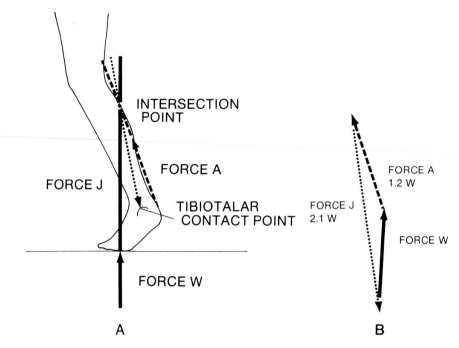

**Figure 6.16.** **A,** On a free body diagram of the foot, including the talus, the lines of application for forces *W* and *A* are extended until they intersect (*intersection point*). The line of application for force *J* is then determined by connecting its point of application (*tibiotalar contact point*) with the intersection point for forces *W* and *A*. **B,** A triangle of forces is constructed. Force *A* is 1.2 times body weight, and force *J* is 2.1 times body weight. (From Frankel V, Nordin M. Basic biomechanics of the skeletal system. Philadelphia: Lea & Febiger, 1980.)

in the maximum voluntary contraction between the anterior tibialis and triceps surae at the extremes of motion. The triceps surae demonstrated a stronger contraction with plantar flexion, and this would be consistent with its function as a static postural muscle. The study did not minimize the effect of the passive restraints and Weiss and co-workers stated that, in quiet standing, the resistance of noncontractile ankle joint tissues to dorsiflexion is significant enough such that only small, periodic bursts of the triceps surae are needed to maintain a stable posture.

## THE FIBULA IN WEIGHT BEARING

The function of the fibula as a weight-bearing structure has been postulated by investigators as its role in the human is known not only as an attachment for ligamentous structures but also as an articulating surface. Lambert (8) used strain gauges in a static mode and estimated the fibula participation in weight bearing to be as much as 16% of the total load. Skraba and Greenwald (18) confirmed this function stating that under physiologic static load testing up to 600 pounds, the fibula bore 15–20% of the applied load. They found a small drop-off in weight bearing after

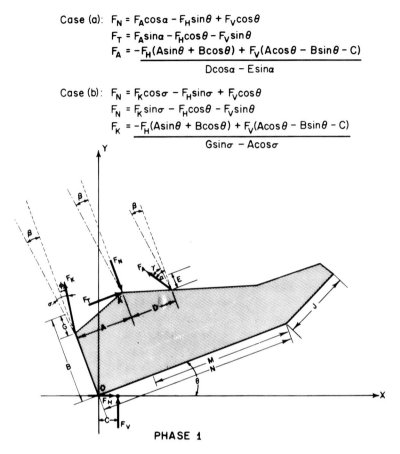

Case (a): $F_N = F_A \cos\alpha - F_H \sin\theta + F_V \cos\theta$

$F_T = F_A \sin\alpha - F_H \cos\theta - F_V \sin\theta$

$$F_A = \frac{-F_H(A\sin\theta + B\cos\theta) + F_V(A\cos\theta - B\sin\theta - C)}{D\cos\alpha - E\sin\alpha}$$

Case (b): $F_N = F_K \cos\sigma - F_H \sin\sigma + F_V \cos\theta$

$F_N = F_K \sin\sigma - F_H \cos\theta - F_V \sin\theta$

$$F_K = \frac{-F_H(A\sin\theta + B\cos\theta) + F_V(A\cos\theta - B\sin\theta - C)}{G\sin\sigma - A\cos\sigma}$$

PHASE 1

**Figure 6.17.** Free-body diagram of the foot during Phase 1 of the stance cycle (heel strike to heel off) and equations derived to solve for compressive force ($F_N$), tangential force ($F_T$), Achilles tendon force ($F_K$), and anterior tibial tendon force. ($F_A$). (From Stauffer R, Chao E, Brewster R. Force and motion analysis of the normal, diseased, and prosthetic ankle joint. Clin Orthop Relat Res 1977;127:190.)

incising the interosseous membrane, suggesting that the support of the fibula may be reduced in this instance. Furthermore, they found an increased load transfer to the fibula with eversion of the ankle complex.

By removing bone and inserting load cells, Takebe et al. (21) used a direct measurement of weight transfer to the fibula. The maximum load transfer measured 6.4% of total load to the lower extremity, but the peak load was only 60 kg. Interestingly, they found increased fibula loading with dorsiflexion and decreased loading with plantar flexion. Also, lateral and posterior loading of the distal tibia increased load transfer to the fibula.

The interosseous membrane plays an important role in the load-sharing ability of the fibula. Minns and Hunter (11) did a strain study of the interosseous membrane,

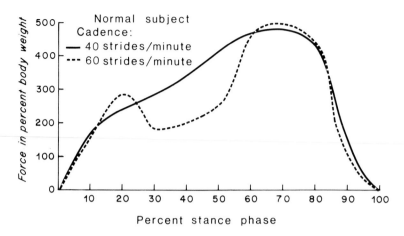

**Figure 6.18.** Effect of varying walking cadence on compressive ankle force ($F_N$). (From Stauffer R, Chao E, Brewster R. Force and motion analysis of the normal, diseased, and prosthetic ankle joint. Clin Orthop Relat Res 1977;127:195.)

demonstrating the ligament can elongate 120% in tension before failure. However, it does not reach full load-carrying capacity until it stretches 50%. The membrane is 45 times stronger in the verticle oblique direction of its fibers than perpendicular to them. Thus, when perpendicular strain is applied to the fibers of the membrane, elongation of more than 300% occurs before failure. This phenomenon allows the membrane to remain intact in tibia fractures. Vukicevic et al. (22) stated that complete damage to the interosseous membrane unburdens the fibula in load transference by more than 30%. Yucel et al. (25) performed a similar study, confirming that the intact interosseous membrane and fibula relieve the tibia by approximately 30%. Skraba and Greenwald (17) indicated that, when the interosseous membrane was cut, fibular strains indicating force transfer dropped to zero. Without the interosseous membrane, the fibula can translate or rotate rather than carry load.

The clinical relevance of the above discussion is to understand the role of the fibula and interosseous membrane in weight bearing, such that in the traumatic condition, their functional loss is recognized. Further study regarding specific strains in these structures should be possible with newer technology.

## MECHANICAL FUNCTION OF LIGAMENTOUS STRUCTURES

The ligaments of the ankle have specific anatomical relationships that allow for normal joint kinematics. Indeed, we measure their importance as suggested by McCullough and Burge (9) who found little change in the function of ligaments even if the articular malleolar surfaces were removed.

**Lateral Ligaments.** The calcaneofibular ligament is an interesting structure in that it effectively spans the ankle and subtalar joints, which have markedly different axes of rotation. This ligament must be attached in such a way as not to restrict motion in either joint, whether they move independently or simultaneously. We see that the origin of the calcaneofibular ligament is the tip of the lateral malleolus, which is at or near the ankle joint axis of rotation. From the tip of the lateral malleolus, the ligament extends obliquely downward and medial to the lateral side of the calcaneus. When projected onto the sagittal plane of the subtalar joint axis, the ligament parallels this axis (Fig. 6.19). When projected onto a vertical transverse plane, the calcaneo-fibular ligament diverges from the subtalar axis at an acute angle (Fig. 6.20).

The motion of the subtalar joint is unlimited, however, as the calcaneofibular ligament lies on the surface of an imaginary cone. The central axis of this imaginary cone is the axis of rotation of the subtalar joint (Fig. 6.21). The angle between the calcaneofibular ligament and the anterior talofibular ligament was measured in two planes on 50 cadaver ankles. The average angles and the distribution of individual values are shown (Fig. 6.22). In the sagittal plane, the angle between the two ligaments may vary from 70 to 140°.

Several points require emphasis. Note that the calcaneofibular ligament retains its parallelism to the axis of the subtalar joint as the ankle passes from plantar flexion to dorsiflexion. In plantar flexion, both the ligament and subtalar joint axis become horizontal, while in dorsiflexion, they approach a more vertical position. Furthermore, in dorsiflexion, the calcaneofibular ligament can act as a true collateral ligament and prevent talar tilt.

The angle between the calcaneofibular ligament and the anterior talofibular lig-ament is approximately 90° in the sagittal plane. As the ankle joint passes from dorsiflexion to plantar flexion, the calcaneofibular ligament is less able to resist talar tilt, and reciprocally, the anterior talofibular ligament is more able to resist talar tilt. Johnson and Markolf (7) studied laxity after sectioning the anterior talofibular liga-

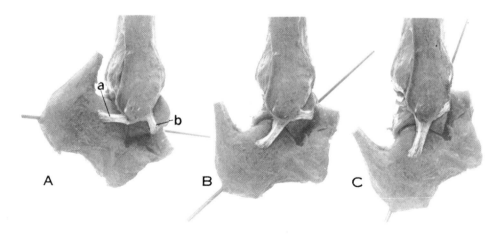

**Figure 6.19.** Dissection of cadaver ankle showing lateral collateral ligaments. The ligaments have been bleached with $H_2O_2$ to increase their contrast. The calcaneofibular ligament (*a*) and the anterior talofibular ligament (*b*) are clearly shown. The posterior talofibular ligament is ob-scured by the overlying fibula. Note the change in positions of the ligaments in relation to the mortise of the ankle joint from full plantar flexion to full dorsiflexion. The angle between the anterior talofibular and calcaneofibular ligaments in this specimen is approximately 125°.

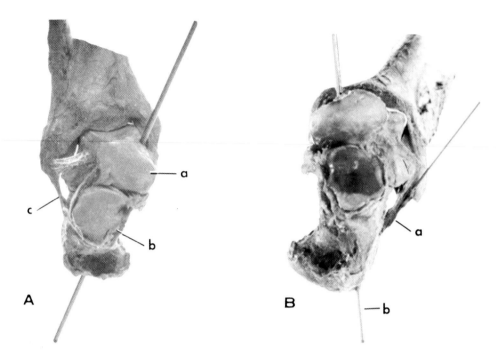

**Figure 6.20.** Cadaver specimen. **A**, Anterior view. In the dissection the entire midfoot and forefoot have been removed. The talus (*a*) is seen articulating in the mortise above and with the calcaneus (*b*) below. The axis of the subtalar joint is represented by the 3-mm rod. The calcaneofibular ligament (*c*) is seen extending from the tip of the lateral malleolus downward and medially to the calcaneus. **B**, Same specimen viewed from below. A Kirschner wire (*a*) has been threaded through the fibers of the calcaneofibular ligament. Note the direction of the ligament extending from the malleolus to the lateral side of the calcaneus. If extended, the Kirschner wire would intersect at an acute angle the axis rod (*b*) within the lateral wall of the calcaneus.

ment and found the most change to occur in plantar flexion. They found a smaller change in laxity in dorsiflexion, suggesting that the anterior talofibular ligament limits talar tilt throughout motion but has greatest advantage in plantar flexion. Rasmussen and Tovborg-Jensen (15) further confirmed the above findings, stating that talar tilt is limited in plantar flexion by the anterior talofibular ligament, in neutral position by the anterior talofibular ligament, and in dorsiflexion by the calcaneofibular ligament plus the posterior talofibular ligament.

Renstrom et al. (16) studied the strain in the two ligaments and found that the anterior talofibular ligament undergoes an increasing strain of 3.3% from 10° of dorsiflexion to 30° of plantar flexion. The calcaneofibular ligament was essentially isometric in the neutral position throughout the flexion arc. The calcaneofibular ligament strain was significantly increased by supination and external rotation. However, with plantar flexion in this position, strain in the calcaneofibular ligament decreased. Thus, this study indicated that the anterior talofibular and calcaneofibular ligaments are synergistic such that when one is relaxed the other is strained. Colville

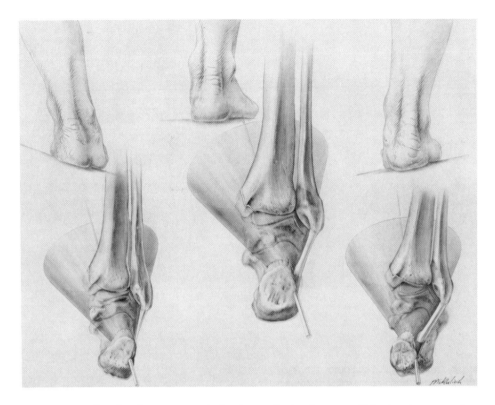

**Figure 6.21.** Functional arrangement of calcaneofibular ligament. This drawing presents a concept that explains the mechanism in which free motion is permitted in the subtalar joint without restriction by the calcaneofibular ligament. An imaginary cone has been drawn around the axis of the subtalar joint. The calcaneofibular ligament is shown converging from its fibular attachment to the calcaneus. Since the ligament lies on the surface of the cone whose apex is the point of intersection of the functional extensions of the ligament and the axis of the subtalar joint, motion of the calcaneus under the talus is allowed without undue restriction from the ligament, which is merely displaced over the surface of the cone.

et al. (2) found similar results using strain gauges on the lateral ligaments. Both the anterior talofibular and calcaneofibular ligaments showed increased strain with ankle inversion. The posterior talofibular ligament demonstrated increased strain in dorsiflexion and external rotation but had minimal resistance to inversion.

**Deltoid Ligament.** Wide variations have been noted in the anatomic description of this structure but we will consider the view of Pankovich, which defines four discrete structures (see Chapter 10). The tibiocalcaneal ligament constitutes the superficial layer of the deltoid and spans the medial malleolus to the medial surface of the calcaneus. The other three divisions, the anterior tibiotalar ligament, intermediate tibiotalar ligament, and posterior tibiotalar ligament, attach the medial malleolus to the talus. The intermediate ligament is "deep" to the tibiocalcaneal ligament, is a very strong ligament, and is only a few millimeters in length.

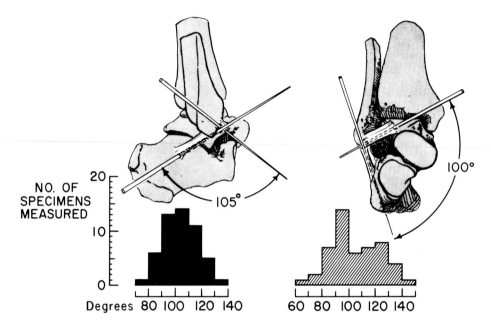

**Figure 6.22.** Average angle between calcaneofibular and talofibular ligaments as measured in sagittal and coronal planes. Note the *histograms*, which indicate a considerable spread (70° in the sagittal and 90° in the coronal plane).

Close (1) found the deltoid ligament to be a strong restraint limiting talar abduction. With all lateral structures removed, he found that the intact deltoid ligament allowed only 2 mm of separation between the talus and medial malleolus. When the "deep" deltoid ligament was incised, the talus could be separated from the medial malleolus by a distance of 3.7 mm. Grath (5) confirmed these findings in a similar experiment. Rasmussen and co-workers (13, 14) investigated the function of various parts of the deltoid ligament and stated that the tibiocalcaneal ligament or "superficial" deltoid specifically limited talar abduction or negative talar tilt. On the other hand, the deep layers of the deltoid ligament rupture in external rotation without the superficial portion being involved.

**Articular Restraints.** From the above discussion, we recognize the importance of the orientation of ligaments and position of the ankle at the time of stress. The third important stabilizing factor is the effect of articular surfaces in providing ankle stability. Fraser and Ahmed (4) demonstrated extensive changes in resistance to axial torque that occurred with compressive loading. In general, loading significantly stabilized the ankle to axial rotation.

Stormont et al. (20) studied the amount of articular stability created after all ligaments were incised. Articular congruity accounted for 30% of the torque resistance to internal and external rotation and virtually 100% of inversion and eversion stability. Michelson (10) studied loaded ankles evaluating talar shift with deltoid ligament sectioning and fibular displacement. He found that lateral fibular displacement did not influence talar shift in the loaded state. The major talar shift occurred when the ankle was taken from the unloaded to the loaded state. However, sectioning the deltoid ligament doubled the average talar shift. This study suggested that the articular surface congruity of ankle joint creates an inherently stable articulation with loading.

**Clinical Relevance.** From the above discussion, we see that the ankle joint is a stable articulation that has both articular and ligament factors influencing stability. In light of recent studies, it is difficult to minimize the value of each in determining clinical outcome of traumatic injury. Consequently, joint stability is the focus of our treatment of these injuries. It is likely that future efforts in clinical research, such as revising existing classification schemes and determining protocols will need primarily to deal with ankle joint stability.

## References

1. Close, J. Some applications of the functional anatomy of the ankle joint. J Bone Joint Surg 1956;38A:761–781.

2. Colville MR, Marder R, Boyle J, Zarins B. Strain measurement in the human ankle ligaments [Abstract]. Orthopaedic Research Society Annual Meeting, Atlanta, Feb. 1988.

3. Frankel V, Nordin M. Basic biomechanics of the skeletal system. Philadelphia: Lea & Febiger, 1980.

4. Fraser B, Ahmed A. Passive rotational stability of the weight-bearing talocrural joint: An invitro biomechanical study. Orthop Trans 1983;7:248.

5. Grath G. Widening of the ankle mortise. A clinical and experimental study. Acta Chir Scand Suppl 1960;263:1–88.

6. Inman VT. The joints of the ankle. Baltimore: Williams & Wilkins, 1976.

7. Johnson JE, Markolf K. The contribution of the anterior talofibular ligament of ankle laxity. J Bone Joint Surg 1983;65A:81–88.

8. Lambert K. The weight-bearing function of the fibula. J Bone Joint Surg 1971;53A:507–513.

9. McCullough C, Burge P. Rotatory stability of the load-bearing ankle. J Bone Joint Surg 1980;62B:460–464.

10. Michelson JD. Effect of loading on tibiotalar alignment. Orthop Res Soc Trans 1990;15:505.

11. Minns R, Hunter J. The mechanical and structural characteristics of the tibio-fibular interosseous membrane. Acta Orthop Scand 1976;47:236–240.

12. Procter P, Paul J. Ankle joint biomechanics. J Biomech 1982;15:627–634.

13. Rasmussen O, Tovborg-Hensen I, Boe S. Distal tibiofibular ligaments, analysis of function. Acta Orthop Scand 1982;53:681–686.

14. Rasmussen O. Stability of the ankle joint. Analysis of the function and traumatology of the ankle ligaments. Acta Orthop Scand Suppl 1985;56: 211:7–72.

15. Rasmussen O, Tovborg-Jensen I. Mobility of the ankle joint. Acta Orthop Scand 1982;53:155–160.

16. Renstrom P, Wertz M, Incavo S, Pope M, Ostgaard C, Arms S, Haugh L. Strain in the lateral ligaments in the ankle [Abstract]. Orthopaedic Research Society Annual Meeting, Atlanta, Feb. 1988.

17. Skraba J, Greenwald A. The role of the interosseous membrane on tibiofibular weightbearing. Foot Ankle 1984;4:301–304.

18. Skraba J, Greenwald A. Weight bearing role of the human fibula. Foot Ankle 1982;2:345–346.

19. Stauffer R, Chao E, Brewster R. Force and motion analysis of the normal, diseased, and prosthetic ankle joint. Clin Orthop Relat Res 1977;127:189–196.

20. Stormont D, Morrey B, Kai-nan A, Cass J. Stability of the loaded ankle: Relation between articular restraint and primary and secondary static restraints. Am J Sports Med 1985;13:295–300.

21. Takebe K, Nakagawa A, Minami H, Kanazawa H, Hirohata K. Role of the fibula in weightbearing. Clin Orthop Relat Res 1984;184:289–292.

22. Vukicevic S, Stern-Padovan R, Vukicevic D, Keros P. Holographic investigations of the human tibiofibular interosseous membrane. Clin Orthop Relat Res 1980;151:210–214.

23. Weiss P, Kearney R, Hunter I. Position dependence of ankle joint dynamics: I. Passive mechanics. J Biomech 1986;19:727–735.

24. Weiss P, Kearney R, Hunter I. Position dependence of ankle joint dynamics: II. Active mechanics. J Biomech 1986;19:737–751.

25. Yucel M, Gadiel H, Scharf H. In vitro-untersuchungen zur tragfunktion der membrana interossea und fibula im hinblick auf die gesamtbelastbarkeit des unterschenkels. Z Orthop 1986;124:273–277.

# 7

# Biomechanics of the Subtalar Joint

BRUCE J. SANGEORZAN, M.D.

The foot has two major functions: support and propulsion. It must be a mobile structure to allow stability on uneven surfaces and a rigid structure to support the body in standing or allow the forefoot to act as a lever in propelling the body forward. The subtalar joint plays a key role in converting the foot from a mobile structure as it must be at heel strike, to a rigid structure as it is at toe off. The subtalar joint also helps the foot to smooth out gait, interface with uneven walking surfaces, act as a shock absorber at heel strike, and extend the extremes of motion of the ankle. Mann (5) called the subtalar joint the "determinative joint of the foot influencing the performance of the more distal articulations and modifying the forces imposed on the skeletal and soft tissues."

Understanding a joint requires that we understand what motion it undergoes, how it distributes weight, and what role it plays in the musculoskeletal system. To understand these phenomena, we measure kinematics (motion) and the joint contact pressures (weight distribution), which are determined by biologically generated forces (muscle), extrinsic forces (gravity), and articular surface orientation. Since the motion is limited by a complex network of ligaments, a basic understanding of their anatomy is necessary as well.

In the case of the talocalcaneal articulation, there are no muscles that originate on one bone and insert on the other. Voluntary motions of the hindfoot are largely determined by muscle tendon units that cross the tibiotalar, talocalcaneal, and transverse tarsal joints and act indirectly on subtalar motion. That fact may enhance the importance of understanding the role of articular surface orientation and contact pressures. Unfortunately, the technology to study these latter parameters has only recently become available. In addition, the subtalar joint has a highly variable shape and motion axis that has defied simple description. Only a small amount of motion occurs in the subtalar joint during straight foreward gait: Wright and Desai (10) measured 6° in neutrally aligned feet. The joint has an axis that indicates it may provide more important function during adaptation to uneven surfaces, turning, or inclines.

## SUBTALAR AXIS AND MOTION

Inman discussed the effect of various theoretical orientations of the subtalar joint on the axis of motion of the subtalar joint. He used a rigid body model with one part representing the foot, one part representing the tibia, and the two connected by a simple hinge. He varied the orientation of that hinge to demonstrate its effect on the direction of motion of the joint. He then discussed the function of the foot-shank complex from each of two reference points: with the foot planted and the leg moving in space, as occurs during stance phase, or with the leg fixed and the foot free. The latter represents a way to better visualize the effect of the axis orientation on the motion of the joint.

With the leg fixed in the vertical axis and the hinge in the sagittal plane of the leg and the midline of the foot, only pure inversion and eversion are allowed (Fig. 7.1). Conversely, if the axis of the subtalar joint, or the hinge, is in the vertical axis, the foot is allowed only a rotatory motion about the vertical axis, which results in adduction or abduction in the horizontal plane (Fig. 7.2). The true subtalar joint axis falls somewhere between these extremes and allows both adduction and abduction as well as inversion and eversion. In a theoretical axis that is located halfway between these two axes, that is forming a 45° angle in the sagittal plane, the amount of inversion and eversion should equal the amount of adduction and abduction (Fig. 7.3). As the axis becomes more horizontal, inversion and eversion will predominate, and as it becomes more vertical, adduction and abduction will predominate. Since there is substantial variation of the axis, between 20° and 57°, the relative motions will vary substantially from person to person. Individuals with flat feet have a subtalar joint

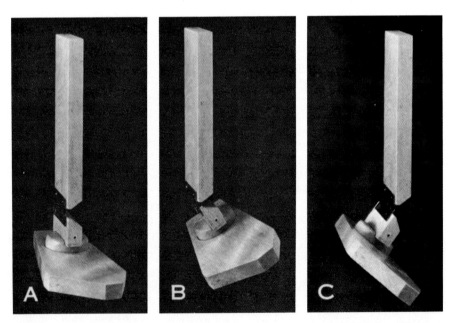

**Figure 7.1.**    Horizontal orientation of axis of subtalar joint (**A**). Note that a horizontal axis permits only inversion (**B**) and eversion (**C**) of the foot.

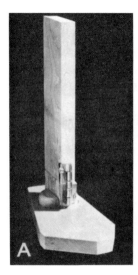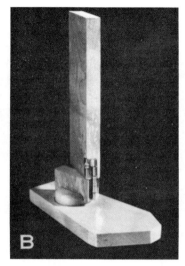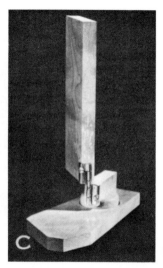

**Figure 7.2.** Vertical orientation of axis of subtalar joint. Note that movement about a vertical axis causes the foot, starting from a neutral position (**A**), to adduct (toe in) (**B**), or to abduct (toe out) (**C**) in the horizontal plane. There is no accompanying eversion or inversion of the foot.

axis that is more horizontal than those with a "neutral" foot. This allows planovalgus feet greater supination and pronation with the same amount of tibial rotation. These people also demonstrate a greater overall range of motion of the subtalar joint (5).

The average axis for the subtalar joint is even more complex since it is not in the sagittal plane of the tibia. It's generally projected medially about 23°. In the studies of Inman, it ranged from 4° to 47°. As this axis deviates medially, the rotation about the axis deviates laterally. The more medial the axis is directed, the larger the component of plantar flexion and dorsiflexion introduced into the motion formula (Fig. 7.4). The described axis demonstrates that the subtalar joint participates in flexion/ extension, inversion/eversion, and adduction/abduction of the foot on the shank.

## Foot Fixed, Leg Free

When the foot is planted on the ground, motion occurs through the ankle and subtalar joint as the leg moves. Any medial, lateral, or anteroposterior motion of the leg upon the foot, because it involves an oblique axis, will introduce some degree of rotation of the leg (Fig. 7.5). The amount of rotation, again, is dependent upon the inclination of the axis of the subtalar joint. If the axis were a pure axis of 45° within the sagittal plane, then 1° of rotation would be accompanied by 1° of angular deviation. As the axis about which the motion occurs becomes more in line with the horizon, the motion about the axis will be relatively more angular and less rotational. As the axis becomes more vertical, a greater amount of rotation will accompany smaller amounts, or rather lesser increments, of angular change (Fig. 7.6). During vigorous activities, such as turning while running, medial and lateral deviation of the leg occurs as well. With more vigorous activities during sports, these angular deviations in the coronal

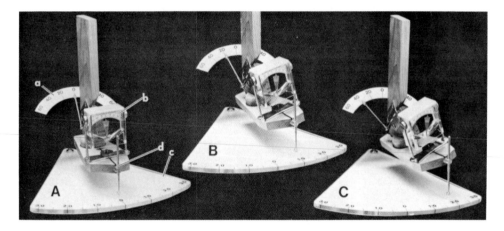

**Figure 7.3.** Subtalar axis inclined to approximate average orientation. In these photographs the hinge connecting the leg and the foot of the model is inclined at 45° (midway between the horizontal, as shown in Fig. 7.1, and the vertical, as shown in Fig. 7.2). Various devices have been added to record angular changes in three planes of space: a goniometer (*a*) indicates actual amount of rotation that occurs in hinge; a Devil Level (*b*), mounted on foot, indicates amount that foot rotates (inverts about its long axis); a horizontal scale (*c*), supported independently, has been placed below the model; a pendulum pointer (*d*) has been attached to the foot. The scale and pointer together, constitute a goniometer that records the amount of adduction (toe-in) that occurs with movement of the subtalar joint. **A**, Neutral position. **B**, Subtalar joint rotated 20°. **C**, Subtalar joint rotated 40° in same direction. Note that a 45° inclination of the axis results in the total amount of movement in the subtalar joint being divided equally between rotation of the foot about its long axis (inversion) and adduction (toe-in). While only inversion and adduction are shown in these photographs, it should be apparent that the same relationships will be obtained when the opposite rotation of the subtalar joint (hinge) occurs.

plane become exaggerated, placing further stresses on the subtalar joint. Without a subtalar joint, this movement could only occur if the foot was not firmly planted, an unstable situation that would clearly diminish our athletic prowess.

### The Subtalar Joint: A Directional Torque Transmitter

Wright and Desai (10) described at length the importance of ankle and subtalar rotation during gait. Inman made the now classical description of the subtalar joint as a torque transmitter. Torque is a force that acts to produce a rotation, and a torque transmitter is a device that applies this rotational force across a joint. Since the pelvis rotates in the horizontal plane as one limb advances in front of the other, and the center of gravity shifts from side to side, some mechanism must exist to allow the bodies to tolerate torsional and angular movement simultaneously (7). Levens et al. (3) found the average rotation of the shank to be about 19° as the body passes over the planted foot. In this circumstance, the plantar surface of the foot is fixed, and rotation and coronal plane angular change is occurring simultaneously. This can occur because of the oblique nature of the ankle and subtalar joint. Although the foot does not slip on the floor, changes do occur within the foot. Rotations that occur in the leg are converted to pronation and supination within the foot (Fig. 7.7). Again, if the

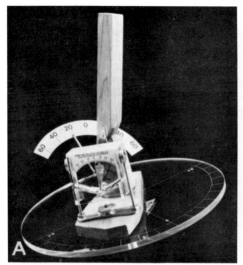
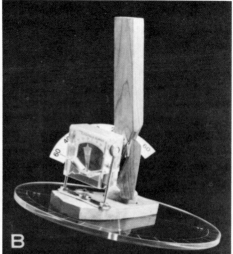

**Figure 7.4.** Effect of posterolateral deviation of axis of subtalar joint from midline of foot. To depict the factor of plantar flexion and dorsiflexion in addition to the previously demonstrated inversion-eversion and adduction-abduction displacements (see Figs. 7.1–7.3), a circular plastic disk has been attached to the foot of the model. The disk has been inscribed in 10° increments, from 0 to 90°. The 0° diameter remains parallel to the anteroposterior plane of the hinge, while the diameters connecting the 90° inscriptions remain perpendicular to the plane of the hinge. The degree of posterolateral deviation of the subtalar joint (hinge) from the midline of the foot can be read from the inscriptions on the disk. Two views only are presented in this figure. In both photographs, the foot has been rotated outward so that the axis of the subtalar joint makes an angle of 40° with the midline of the foot. Note that, in **A**, motion of 20° in the subtalar joint causes the foot to invert and adduct as previously demonstrated but also imposes a degree of plantar flexion. In **B,** the reverse displacements are shown.

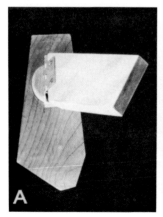
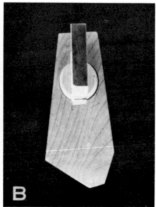
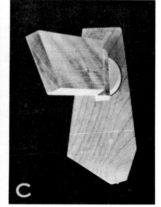

**Figure 7.5.** Movement of subtalar joint with foot immobilized. The model demonstrates clearly that, with a fixed foot, motion in the subtalar joint can occur only through lateral or medial deviation of the leg. In these photographs, the subtalar axis is inclined 45°. This inclination imposes longitudinal rotations of the leg, which must accompany the lateral and medial deviations.

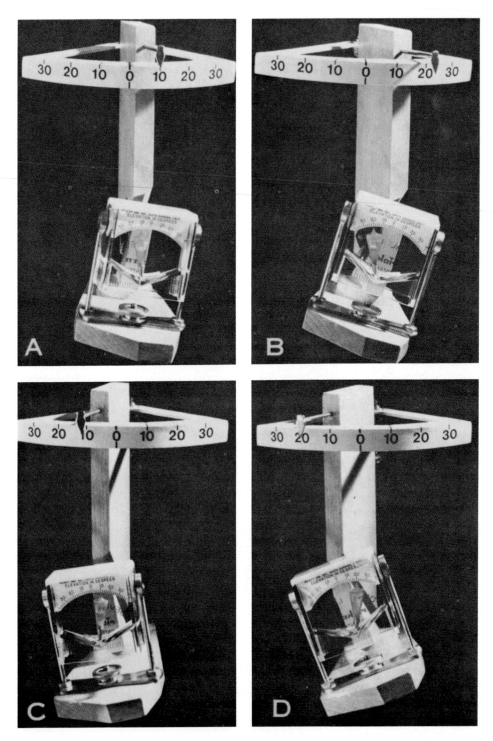

**Figure 7.6.** Relationship between rotation of leg and pronation-supination of foot. Medial rotation of the leg is shown in **A** and **B**. Note that the foot pronates an equal amount as indicated by the Devil Level. Lateral rotation is shown in **C** and **D**. Note that the foot supinates the same amount. This equality in angular displacements exists only if the subtalar axis is inclined at 45°.

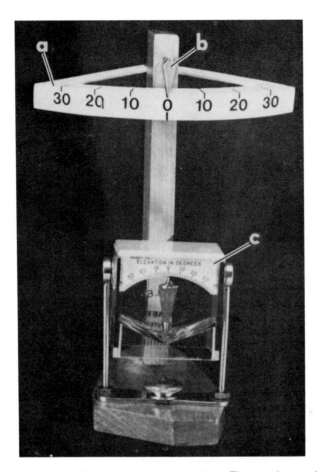

**Figure 7.7.** Subtalar joint as directional torque transmitter. The wooden model selected has the subtalar axis oriented at 45° to the horizontal and in line with the midline of the foot. It is mounted so that the vertical member representing the leg remains vertical but can be rotated in a transverse plane about its long axis. A scale (a) is supported independently of the model. A pointer (b) is attached to the vertical member: a and b constitute a goniometer that records the amount of internal and external rotation of the leg. The foot will remain in the sagittal plane but can rotate about a horizontal axis (pronate or supinate). The degree of pronation or supination is recorded by the Devil Level (c).

axis of inclination of the joint were to be fixed at 45°, an equal amount of pronation and supination would occur with equal amounts of internal and external rotation. As the axis becomes more vertical, less and less supination and pronation occur. As the axis becomes more horizontal, a greater amount of rotation is needed to bring about any pronation in the foot.

Attempts have been made to correlate the amount of supination to the amount of internal outward rotation of the tibia. Olerud and Rosendahl (6) found a linear relationship with 0.44° of external tibial rotation for each degree of supination of the foot. However, others (1) have found that average values of the hindfoot are of little value because of the great amount of variation.

Wright and Desai (10) studied changes in the ankle and subtalar movement with in-toeing and out-toeing. With the toes turned in during gait, there was a relative increase in the amount of rotation in the subtalar joint and a relative decrease in angular displacement in the ankle joint, when compared with normal gait in the same individual period. Toeing out appeared to have a less dramatic impact on subtalar rotation with slightly greater supination from heel-rise to toe-off.

## Contact Pressures

Contact pressure in the talocalcaneal joint of cadaver specimens has been investigated recently using pressure-sensitive film. The contact pressures were studied in varus, neutral, and valgus alignment at multiple applied loads. Contact pressures and surface areas of contact within the subtalar joint occur in increasing amounts with increasing load. The location of the contact area does not change with inversion and eversion of the foot, although the overall contact area shows a progressive increase with increasing load. At any applied load, the inverted foot has smaller contact area with greater overall average pressure than the neutral or everted foot. No statistical difference in contact area or pressures occurred between neutral and valgus alignment. This information supports the clinical observation that varus hindfoot alignment is poorly tolerated and leads to early degenerative changes.

## Pathologic Circumstances

The subtalar joint also plays a compensatory role in diminishing the impact of angular deformity. The subtalar joint is particularly suited to this task when the deformities are varus or valgus but somewhat less suited for flexion and extension deformities of the tibia. When motion is lost in the subtalar joint, the tibiotalar joint loses it's ability to compensate for angular deformity in the coronal plane (9).

Alignment of the hindfoot must be maintained during any surgical arthrodesis. An ankle arthrodesis should be a neutral dorsiflexion and plantar flexion, 0–5° of valgus, and an equal or slightly greater amount of external rotation when compared to the opposite limb. A similar attempt at maintaining a neutral position should be followed in a subtalar or triple arthrodesis. In another study, Lundberg and Svensson (4) studied the influence of pronation and supination using stereophotogrammetry and found that the tibia showed an average of 0.2° of external rotation for each degree of supination. In this study, the greatest movement during supination occurred at the talonavicular joint, and somewhat less occurred at the talocalcaneal joint.

Siegler et al. (8) studied cadaver motion in freshly amputated specimens. The most important finding was that the range of motion of the foot-shank complex in any direction is larger than that of either the ankle or subtalar joints alone. This means that the subtalar joint contributes in a small way to dorsiflexion and plantar flexion, and in a larger fashion to inversion and eversion. Internal and external rotation of the foot-shank complex occurs at both the ankle and subtalar joints more than previously realized. Engsberg et al. (2) attempted to predict the position of the talus relative to the calcaneus based on the position of the shank to the calcaneus. This relatively logical prediction was based upon the fact that the talus has no tendon insertions and its position should be passively determined by forces acting across the ankle and subtalar joint. However, the authors found that significant variations within and between specimens largely limited predictive value. They also found that adduction orientations were much better predictors than were eversion/inversion orientations and suggested that foot categories be developed based on the orientation of these joints.

## SUMMARY

The subtalar joint acts as a mitered hinge. A mitered hinge functions as a directional torque transmitter. Forces acting to induce a rotation about the longitudinal axis of the tibia are transmitted to torques about the longitudinal axis of the foot, i.e., supination and pronation. The reverse is true as well. Rotational torques induced by the foot are transmitted as a rotational torque about the tibia. Pronation is defined as external rotation of the foot relative to the tibia combined with hindfoot eversion, combined with outward rotation of the foot on its own longitudinal axis. Supination describes an internal rotation of the foot on the tibia combined with hindfood inversion and a converse rotation of the foot about its own longitudinal axis. When the foot pronates, the tibia is internally rotated; when it supinates the tibia is externally rotated.

### References

1. Engsberg JR. A biomechanical analysis of the talocalcaneal joint — In vitro. J Biomech 1987;20:429–442.
2. Engsberg JR, Grimston SK, Wackwitz JH. Predicting talocalcaneal joint orientations from talocalcaneal/talocrural joint orientations. J Orthop Res 1988;6(5):749–757.
3. Levens AS, Inman VT, Blosser JA. Transverse rotation of segments, lower extremity and locomotion. J Bone Joint Surg 1948;30A:859.
4. Lundberg A, Svensson OK, Bylund C, Goldie I, Selvik G. Kinematics of the ankle/foot complex. Part II: Pronation and supination. Foot Ankle 1989;9:248–253.
5. Mann RA. Biomechanics of the foot and ankle. In: Mann RA, ed. Surgery of the foot. 5th ed. Toronto: CV Mosby, 1986:1–31.
6. Olerud C, Rosendahl Y. Torsion transmitting properties of the hindfoot. Curr. Orthop. Relat. Res. 1987;214:285–294.
7. Saunders JB, deCM, Inman VT, Eberhart HB. The major determinants in normal and pathologic gait. J Bone Joint Surg 1953;35A:543.
8. Siegler S, Chen J, Schenck CD. The three dimensional kinematics and flexibility characteristics of the human ankle and subtalar joint. Part I: Kinematics. J Biomech Eng 1988;110:364–373.
9. Ting A, Tarr RR, Sarmiento A, Wagner K, Resnick C. The role of subtalar motion and ankle contact, pressure changes from angular deformities of the tibia. Foot Ankle 1987;7:290–299.
10. Wright DG, Desai SM, Henderson WH. Action of the subtalar and ankle joint complex during the stance phase of walking. J Bone Joint Surg 1964;46A:361.

# 8

# Analysis of Ankle and Subtalar Motion during Human Locomotion

GERALD F. HARRIS, Ph.D

The process of normal ambulation requires that the foot and ankle participate in the kinematic and kinetic events associated with lower extremity motion and load bearing. As an integrated mechanism, the ankle and subtalar joints work in unison to provide a smooth transition of forces. The fascinating sequence of events required for this even transition extends well beyond the commonly observed sagittal motion patterns of ankle dorsiflexion and plantar flexion.

To better understand ankle and subtalar joint function, we should visualize several rotations occurring simultaneously in the leg and foot. The ankle joint has an oblique axis in the frontal plane, rotated laterally downward 82.0° (±3.6°) from tibial midline (Fig. 8.1). In the transverse plane, the axis is laterally and posteriorly directed 20–30° (Fig. 8.2). As a result of these oblique axes, the foot externally rotates when the ankle is in maximum dorsiflexion. When maximally plantar flexed, the foot internally rotates. During the stance phase of gait, the foot is fixed to the ground surface, resulting in internal rotation of the tibia with ankle dorsiflexion and external tibial rotation with ankle plantar flexion. These rotations are independent of subtalar motion.

The subtalar joint has been described by Close and Inman as a mitered hinge as illustrated in Figure 8.3 (2). If the hinge axis is at 45°, rotation of the vertical member results in equal rotation of the horizontal member. Changing the hinge axis to a more horizontal orientation causes a larger rotation of the horizontal member for the same vertical member rotation. The opposite is true if the hinge axis is more vertically placed. The subtalar joint axis measures 42° (±9°) from horizontal in the sagittal plane and 23° (±11°) from foot midline in the transverse plane (8) (Fig. 8.4).

A closer approximation to the true anatomic relationship is illustrated in Figure 8.5 in which the motion of the talonavicular joint is included. This model of talocalcaneal navicular motion was developed by Inman and co-workers (6, 7). The distal horizontal member consists of two structures: a medial representation of the three medial rays of the foot and a lateral representation of the two lateral rays. The model helps explain the observation of external rotation of the leg, resulting in supination of the foot, and internal rotation, resulting in pronation of the foot. During gait, external rotation of the leg results in forefoot supination, which is followed by a

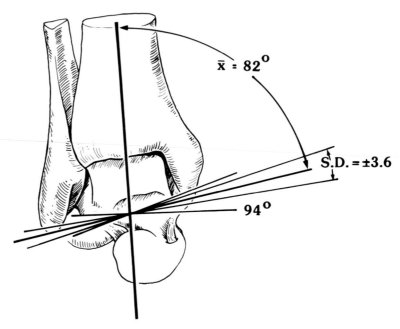

**Figure 8.1.**   The ankle joint axis with reference to the tibial midline.

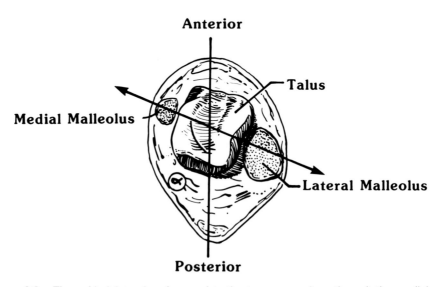

**Figure 8.2.**   The ankle joint axis referenced to the transverse plane through the medial and lateral malleoli. Angle $\alpha$ is the angle of the axis to the anterior-posterior plane, 110–120°. (Adapted from Tylkowski CM. Lovell & Winter's pediatric orthopaedics. Philadelphia: JB Lippincott, 1990.)

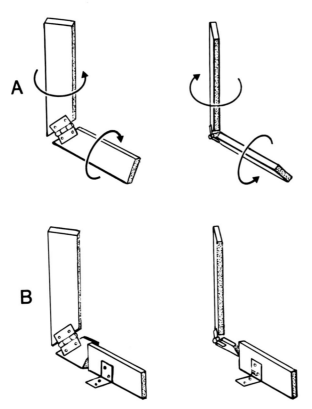

**Figure 8.3.** The mitered hinge mechanism demonstrating rotational relationships. **A,** Simple hinge motion. **B,** Addition of a pivot between the hinged segments. (Adapted from Mann RA. Surgery of the foot. St. Louis: CV Mosby, 1986.)

pronation twist of the foot to remain plantigrade. As a result of these motions, the foot tends to mechanically lock, acting as a rigid body. With internal leg rotation, the opposite sequence of events takes place tending to mechanically unlock the foot.

During ambulation, stance and swing phase events occur in an orderly sequence to allow weight transition, energy transfer, and smooth motion progression. The events occurring within these phases include three intervals for stance and one for swing. The stance events include double limb support (during 0–12% of the gait cycle), single limb support (during 12–50% of the gait cycle), and a final stance period of double limb support (50–65% of the gait cycle). Swing phase accounts for the remaining 45% of the gait cycle.

Initial double limb support begins with heel strike and rapid plantar flexion of the ankle from an initial position of slight dorsiflexion (Fig. 8.6). As the foot is loaded, pronation occurs, which, according to Mann, is a passive structural mechanism (7). With foot pronation, the leg rotates internally as a direct result of the subtalar linkage between leg and foot. Electromyographic activity during the initial phase is limited to that of the tibialis anterior (9) (Fig. 8.7).

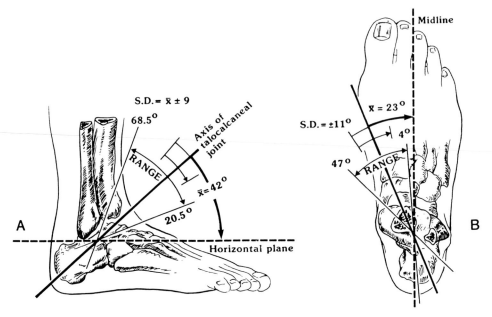

**Figure 8.4.** The subtalar joint axes with reference to A. sagittal plane orientation (**A**) and transverse plane orientation (**B**). (Adapted from Inman VT. The joints of the ankle. Baltimore: Williams & Wilkins, 1976.)

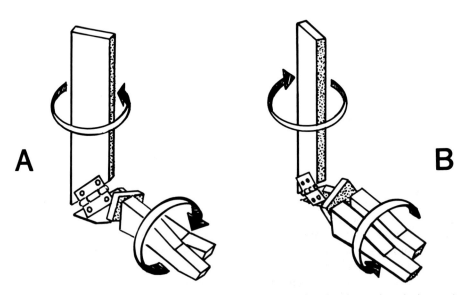

**Figure 8.5.** The mitered hinge mechanism altered to include talocalcaneal navicular motion. (Adapted from Mann RA. Surgery of the foot. St. Louis: CV Mosby, 1986.)

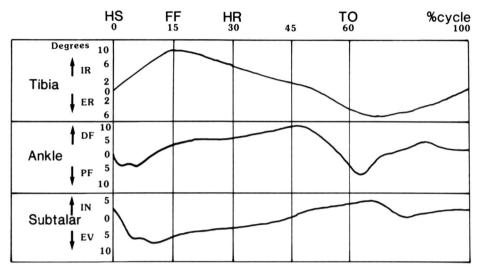

**Figure 8.6.** Tibial, ankle, and subtalar motion referenced to foot contact events. (Adapted from Sarraphian SK. Anatomy of the foot and ankle. Philadelphia: JB Lippincott, 1983.)

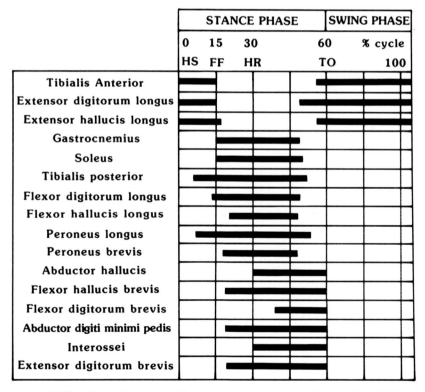

**Figure 8.7.** EMG activity of the leg and foot muscles during normal ambulation. (Adapted from Tylkowski CM. Lovell & Winter's pediatric orthopaedics, Philadelphia: JB Lippincott, 1990.)

During the second stance interval (single limb support), the center of gravity of the body passes over the weight-bearing leg while the foot remains flat and immobile on the walking surface. Dorsiflexion of the ankle occurs, accompanied by external tibial rotation and a volley of simultaneous muscular activity (Fig. 8.7). The combined action of the muscles results in hindfoot and midfoot inversion accompanied by external rotation of the leg. Electromyographic (EMG) activity during the second stance phase is seen in the gastrocnemius-soleus, posterior tibialis, peroneal, and toe flexor muscles (9).

The third and final stance interval (double limb support) is characterized by rapid plantar flexion of the ankle, foot supination, and external rotation of the leg. Foot intrinsic and tibialis posterior EMG activity is seen during this phase as the foot acts

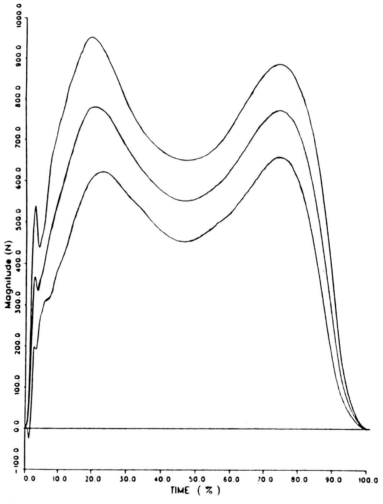

**Figure 8.8.** Averaged vertical component of the barefoot ground reaction force recorded for left foot strike from normal adult males. The mean value is bracketed by one standard deviation.

as a rigid lever during toe off (9). Dorsiflexion of the toes aids in stabilizing the arch of the foot through the windlass mechanism of Hicks (5). The plantar aponeurosis shortens with extension of the metatarsophalangeal joints, causing elevation of the arch, passive inversion of the heel, and greater stability.

The swing phase is characterized by ankle dorsiflexion, neutral subtalar position, and contraction of the tibialis anterior.

Insight into the ground reaction forces of foot to floor contact during gait may be gained by inspecting the output from a force dynamometer imbedded within the laboratory walkway. Such systems typically record vertical and shear forces as well as the moment of force about the vertical axis (3, 4). An illustration of the vertical ground reaction force taken from 10 normal adults is provided in Figure 8.8. Upon foot

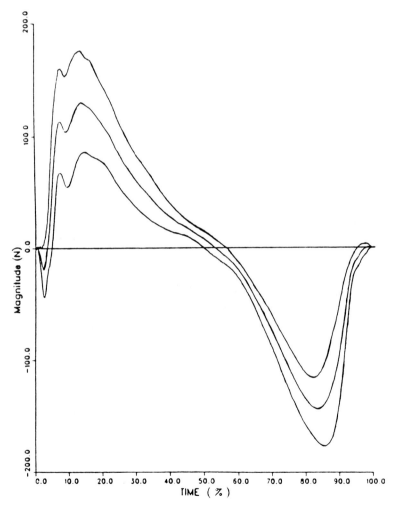

**Figure 8.9.** Averaged fore/aft shear component of the barefoot ground reaction force recorded for left foot strike from 10 normal adult males. The mean value is bracketed by one standard deviation.

strike, the vertical force rises quickly to an initial peak value of 40–60% body weight, followed more slowly by a rise to between 100 and 120% of body weight. This initial region of the curve is called the loading portion. A gradual decline in vertical force to values less than body weight is then observed with the minimum occurring near the center of the single limb support phase. The weight reduction seen during this portion of the curve occurs as the body center of mass moves vertically over the supporting foot. With preparation for opposite foot strike, the vertical force rises once again to a second peak and then rapidly diminishes with initiation of swing phase.

An illustration of fore/aft shear is depicted in Figure 8.9. Following a brief aft

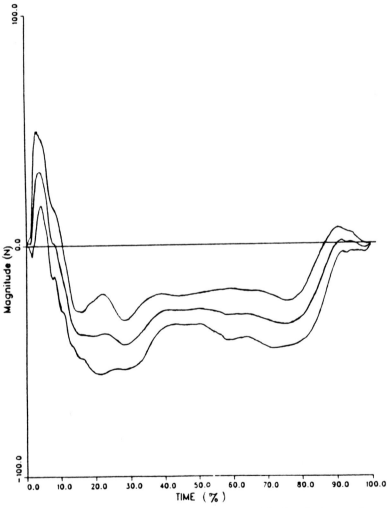

**Figure 8.10.** Averaged medial lateral shear component of the barefoot ground reaction force recorded for left foot strike from 10 normal adult males. The mean value is bracketed by one standard deviation.

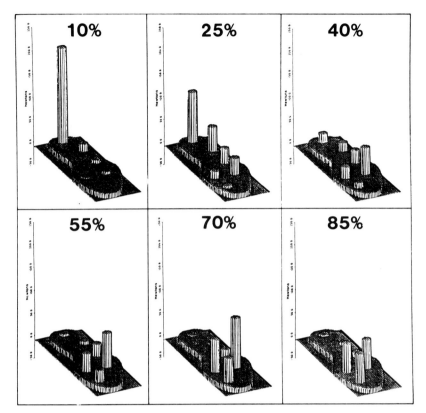

**Figure 8.11.** Foot contact force sequence illustrating the progression of force transition from heel strike through stance. Data represent average values for a sample of 10 normal adult males.

shear with initial foot contact, forward shear proceeds, increasing rapidly until opposite toe off, and then decreasing to zero near midstance. With direction reversal, an aft shear peak is noted near the time of opposite foot strike.

A much smaller medial/lateral shear is seen in gait (Fig. 8.10). A brief, rapid initial medial peak is seen probably representing the hip adduction of the lower extremity at foot strike. The lateral shear that follows is due to the medial location of the body center of mass over the center of pressure.

A summary of results from a vertical force analysis of discrete pressure components during stance is depicted in Figure 8.11 for a portable force dosimeter system using six integral sensors mounted in the sole of a tennis shoe (1, 10). This series illustrates changes in vertical force distribution as stance progresses from heel strike through load acceptance, unloading, and toe off at 15% cycle intervals.

### References

1. Acharya KR, Harris GF, Riedel SA, Kazarian L. Force magnitude and spectral frequency content of heel strike during gait. Proc IEEE Eng Med Biol Soc, 1989: 826–827.

2. Close JR, Inman VT, Poor PM, Todd FN. The function of the subtalar joint. Clin Orthop Relat Res 1967; 50:159–179.

3. Harris GF. Quantitative methods for the eval-

uation of patients with cerebral palsy [Dissertation]. Milwaukee, WI: Marquette University, 1981:451.

4. Harris GF, Salamon NJ, Weber RC. Effect of subject position on balance platform measurements. Trans ASME J Biomech Eng 1981;103:213–216.

5. Hicks JH. The foot as a support. Acta Anat 1955;25:34.

6. Inman VT, Ralston HJ, Todd FL. Human walking. Baltimore: Williams & Wilkins, 1981.

7. Mann RA. Biomechanics of the foot and ankle. In: Mann RA, ed. Surgery of the foot. 5th ed. St. Louis: CV Mosby, 1986:1–30.

8. Sarrafian K. Anatomy of the foot and ankle. Philadelphia: JB Lippincott, 1983.

9. Tylkowski CM. Assessment of gait in children and adolescents. In: Morrissy RT, ed. Lovell and Winter's pediatric orthopaedics. 3rd ed. Philadelphia: JB Lippincott, 1990:57–90.

10. Zhu H, Harris GF, Wertsch J. A microprocessor based data acquisition system for measuring plantar pressure distribution in ambulatory subjects. IEEE Trans Biomed Eng, in press.

# 9

# Applications to Ankle Trauma and Areas of Future Clinical Research

## ARSEN M. PANKOVICH, M.D.

### HISTORICAL OVERVIEW

Fractures of the ankle have intrigued surgeons for at least the last two centuries. Much effort has been devoted to advancing our understanding of the anatomy and function of the ankle joint and to improving treatment methods of ankle fractures. As we shall see, classifying the mechanisms of injuries has been a major focus, and most authors have tried to determine how each fracture occurs. Obviously, our knowledge has evolved greatly over the years to the present understanding that multiple forces and positions of the foot and ankle are likely to combine and cause recognized injury patterns.

Perhaps the most fascinating historical account of ankle fractures is found in an extensive treatise by Ashhurst and Bromer (1). They reviewed every publication that had been written on the subject, and particularly the ankle literature of the 19th century. One can find all varieties of supination-external rotation lesions, fractures of the fibula with tibial substitution, and a rare type known as dislocation of the fibula behind the tibia with a fracture of the fibula in its upper third, which they attributed to Huguier, whereas Bosworth (3) described the same lesion with a low fracture of the fibula. Bonnin (2) stated that simplicity in classification of ankle fractures is not a scientific goal and that the investigators of the subject must realize that they are facing a rather complicated material to be classified. His monograph "Injuries of the Ankle" made a profound impression on clinicians at the time and, needless to say, left them with a complex scheme of classification.

Honigschmied (7) had made an impressive series of experiments in cadavers and accurately described lesions produced by different mechanisms of injury. Recently, Rasmussen (15) reported on an extensive study on ankles in cadavers in which function and vulnerability of ankle ligaments were examined and their relation to stability of the ankle determined. Although every possible motion and combination of motions was tested, many of resulting injuries probably never occur in vivo. Thus, rupture of the calcaneofibular ligament, with intact anterior talofibular ligament, never occurred in my experience nor according to Brostrom (4) and Lindstrand (10), who reported on operative findings in ankle sprains. In my experience, injuries of the anterior talofibular and calcaneofibular ligaments are extremely rare in combination with typical external rotation fractures. I have seen only a few cases of rupture of the anterior talofibular ligament associated with these fractures, and then always in cases with extensive soft tissue injury.

The experimental work of Lauge-Hansen (9) brought about a logical classification of ankle injuries based on mechanisms of the injuries and their consequent anatomic lesions. However accurate the described mechanisms and their anatomic lesions, many already well-described lesions were not covered by Lauge-Hansen's classification. Thus, missing were a variety of fractures above the syndesmosis including Maisonneuve lesions, fractures below the syndesmosis of external rotation type with frequently associated Wagstaffe fracture, Nelaton-Bosworth dislocations, and a variety of injuries of the lateral collateral ligamentous complexes and their associated lesions. Despite these shortcomings, this classification has left a lasting impression on present day orthopaedic surgeons, much as those previous authors had in their day.

## CURRENT CONCEPTS ON ANKLE FRACTURES

After having reviewed the literature and some 1500 ankle injuries from my own experience and having done a limited number of experiments on cadavers, I have extended the Lauge-Hansen classification to include lesions already described in the literature plus some of my own.

It must be understood that each described position of the ankle is not a fixed position or extreme position. Rather, I would suggest a variety of positions, for example, from extreme foot supination through neutral to extreme pronation. Furthermore, the degree of supination or pronation may be changing while the injuring force is acting on the ankle. Likewise, the intensity of the force can change during this time. Though it is convenient to speak of foot and ankle position during the injury event, I believe we must consider a dynamic process of changing positions of the ankle joint combined with changing forces acting on it. Only with such a view in mind, can we explain a great variety of patterns in ankle fractures.

The question of ankle stability is often raised. What constitutes an unstable ankle? Obviously, rupture of any ligament of the ankle will render the talus unstable in certain positions, and so will any fracture. Yet, for practical purposes, the ankle is diagnosed unstable when the talus is displaced or displaceable within the mortise: (a) in lateral direction, indicating rupture of the deep deltoid ligament or a fracture of the medial malleolus along with a fracture of the fibula, or (b) in anteroposterior direction, either from rupture of the anterior talofibular and calcaneofibular ligaments, or a fracture of the posterior tibial tubercle or process, or rupture of the posterior talofibular ligament.

The following short review of ankle fractures is not intended to discuss the classification in detail. All ankle lesions, as encountered in my series and correlated with the data in the literature, are presented in Figures 9.1 and in 9.2. Various stages of these lesions have been described previously. I would like to point out certain findings that have increased my understanding of these injuries.

It is clear from the literature that supination-external rotation (SE) fractures occur

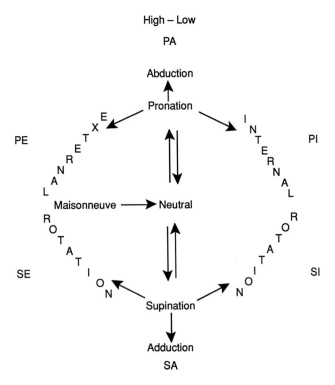

**Figure 9.1.**   Classification of ankle fractures. Different types are shown according to the position of the foot (pronation, neutral, and supination) and the direction of the force (abduction, adduction, internal and external rotation). SE lesions of the fibula occur above, at, and below the syndesmosis. SE lesions below the syndesmosis often contain a Wagstaffe fracture; those at the syndesmosis rarely result in Nelaton-Bosworth dislocation. Other factors that influence formation of fracture types are: ligamentous laxity or rigidity, bone quality (normal or osteoporotic), and foot position (dorsiflexion, plantar flexion).

at three levels along the fibula: at, above, and below the syndesmosis. Lauge-Hansen (9) described the SE fracture of the fibula only at the level of the syndesmosis. He believed, as do a number of contemporary authors, that all fractures of the fibula above the syndesmosis are actually pronation-external rotation (PE) lesions. That this is not the case indicates existence of at least three types of fractures at that level: SE, PE, and PA (pronation-abduction) (11). The existence of SE fractures above the syndesmosis was shown in patients who had no medial tenderness and had neither a fracture of the medial malleolus nor a rupture of the deltoid ligament, as demonstrated by a negative external rotation stress roentgenogram, although these medial lesions would be the initial stage in a PE-type fracture. The existence of PA fractures of the fibula above the syndesmosis is evident from the cases in which the medial side of the ankle is injured, most often by rupture of the deltoid ligament, with a coexisting complete diastasis of the syndesmosis, including the anterior and posterior tibiofibular ligamentous complexes, the interosseous ligament, and often the interosseous mem-

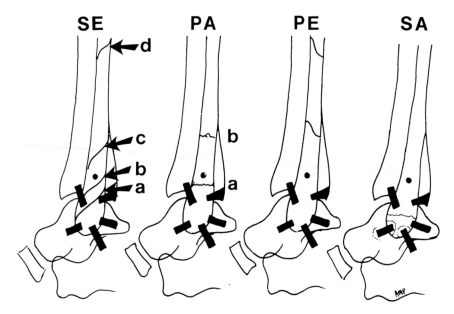

**Figure 9.2.** Different fracture types at different levels along the fibula. The ligaments are shown intact, though are ruptured in many lesions. I, *SE* lesions: The deep deltoid ligament or the medial malleolus are injured as the last stage of an SE lesion. *a*, Mixed oblique fracture of Destot; the anterior tibiofibular ligament is intact in most cases. *b*, Fracture at the syndesmosis; both anterior and posterior tibiofibular ligament complexes are injured in complete lesions. *c*, Fracture above the syndesmosis; the interosseous ligament is also ruptured. *d*, Maisonneuve fracture. II, *PA* lesions: The medial malleolus-deltoid complex and the syndesmosis are always injured before the fibula. *a*, Low PA; the fibular fracture is at the level of the syndesmosis and the interosseous ligament is most often intact while the tibiofibular ligaments are ruptured. *b*, high PA; the interosseous ligament and the membrane are also ruptured. III, *PE* lesions: The medial malleolus-deltoid complex and the anterior tibiofibular and interosseous complexes are injured before the fibula. The last to be injured is the posterior tibiofibular complex. PE-Maisonneuve fracture develops the same as the SE lesion where the fibula fractures before the medial malleolus-deltoid complex is injured. IV, *SA* lesions: Either the medial malleolus fractures first, or the fibula or collateral ligaments are injured first, or they follow each other in combined lesions.

brane. This does not follow the pattern of a PE lesion in which the posterior tibiofibular ligamentous complex is disrupted only after the fracture of the fibula has occurred.

The SE fracture of the fibula below the syndesmosis, the so-called mixed oblique fracture of Destot, is quite often associated with a type-2 Wagstaffe fracture (12, 17). It is produced when the externally rotating talus breaks off the anterior end of the proximal fragment, which, in these low fractures, represents the anterior fibular tubercle protruding below the level of the plafond.

The pronation-internal rotation (PI) mechanism is probably responsible for rupture of the anterior talofibular ligament in an isolated injury. In studies on cadavers, I have observed that the anterior talofibular ligament is taut, while all other ligaments are lax, when internal rotation is applied on a pronated foot. Honigschmied (7) showed frequent rupture of the anterior talofibular ligament in experiments on cadavers when applying internal rotation force. However, he did not indicate the position of the foot. This mechanism may be operative even when plantar flexion of the foot is a part of the injurying mechanism. Lauge-Hansen (9) produced a fracture of the tibia by this mechanism. Rasmussen (15) also tested the combinations of plantar flexion, dorsiflexion, and neutral position with internal rotation. Common injury was a rupture of the anterior talofibular ligament in the first stage, although other ligamentous ruptures followed. Inman (8) favored inversion and plantar flexion as a mechanism of injury of the anterior talofibular ligament, because it is taut in that position while the calcaneofibular ligament is more horizontal and less vulnerable to the talar tilt.

Supination-internal rotation (SI) mechanism is thought to be operative in injuries of the lateral collateral ligaments, in my view probably of both the anterior talofibular and calcaneofibular ligaments. The ligaments are taut when internal rotation force is applied on a supinated foot. In addition, I have seen a number of cases in which a transverse or slightly oblique, and often spiral, fracture of the medial malleolus is accompanied with ruptures of the lateral collateral ligaments. This should be kept in mind when such a fracture of the medial malleolus is encountered.

In the classical view, there are two lesions on the medial side of the ankle: fracture of the medial malleolus and rupture of the deltoid ligament. Not generally understood is the fact that the main stabilizer of the ankle is the deep portion of the deltoid ligament, which is attached posteriorly on the medial malleolus. Close (6) described the deep deltoid ligament and its function very well.

In studies on cadavers, I have found that the three parts of the superficial deltoid ligament are attached to the anterior colliculus (13) (Figs. 9.3, A and B). They reinforce the capsule but are not situated within the joint. On the other hand, the deep deltoid ligament is an intraarticular structure and is attached to the posterior colliculus and the intercollicular groove (Fig. 9.4, A and B). This part is further covered by the overlying posterior tibialis tendon.

There are several important injuries on the medial side of the ankle (14). An isolated fracture of the anterior colliculus leaves the deep deltoid ligament intact, as it is attached to the posterior colliculus (Fig. 9.5, A and B). The mechanism of avulsion of the anterior colliculus appears to be tension on the superficial deltoid, which occurs in forced external rotation. The talus is stable in the mortise, and the commonly associated SE fracture of the fibula is unlikely to be displaced. However, ankle stability must be tested further by external rotation stress roentgenograms, in order to exclude a concurrent rupture of the deep deltoid ligament (Fig. 9.5B). In cases in which there are concurrent lesions (Fig. 9.6), fixation of the anterior collicular fracture does not stabilize the talus, and its lateral shift is still possible. Buttressing of the talus, by fixation of the fibular fracture, retains it undisplaced and allows healing of the deep deltoid ligament.

Fracture of the posterior colliculus, which is often recognized by a supramalleolar spike (Fig. 9.7), remains attached to the deep deltoid ligament and is rarely displaced because the posterior tibial tendon, which passes in its posterior groove, tends to push the fragment back to its place. Roentgenograms of the ankle in 20° of external rotation show clearly the fragment (Fig. 9.8).

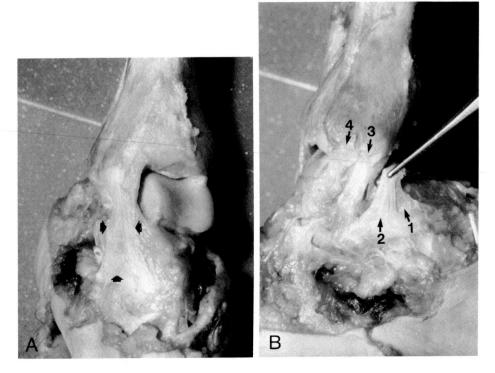

**Figure 9.3.** The superficial portion of the deltoid ligament takes origin from the anterior colliculus. **A,** The naviculotibial ligament (*arrows*). **B,** Detached from the anterior colliculus are: naviculotibial (*1*) and calcaneofibular (*2*) ligaments; still attached is the superficial talotibial ligament (*3*). In view is also the deep posterior talotibial ligament (*4*). (From Pankovich AM, Shivaram MS. Anatomical basis of variability in injuries of the medial malleolus and the deltoid ligament. I. Anatomical studies. Acta Orthop Scand 1979;50:221.)

In my experience, an isolated rupture of the deltoid ligament does not exist, and, if it does occur, it is difficult to recognize it. If left untreated, it does not produce a permanent ankle instability. Cedell (5) described four cases in which the deep deltoid (posterior deep talotibial) ligament avulsed a bone fragment from the talus. In my view, the deep deltoid ligament needs no repair in these lesions provided the syndesmosis is stable.

Diagnosis of a rupture of the deep deltoid ligament is often quite easy. The problem has been how to measure lateral displacement of the talus. I have studied 20 volunteers with normal ankles. A mortise view was obtained of both ankles, then an external rotation stress roentgenogram. This study was designed to determine normal variations of talar displacement with stress and to find the best way to measure the increase in the medial clear space. It became clear that in normal ankles only the superior clear space was of the same width when measured between the junction of the medial malleolus and the plafond and the lateral border of the talus and the plafond (Fig. 9.9). On stress roentgenograms, the difference in width between the

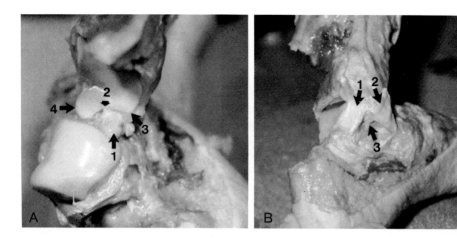

**Figure 9.4.**   The deep portion of the deltoid ligament **A,** Lateral (intraarticular) view of the deep posterior talotibial ligament and its attachments to the talus (*1*), the intercollicular groove (*2*), and the posterior colliculus (*3*). The anterior colliculus (*4*) has a few ligamentous attachments. **B,** Medial view of the deep posterior talotibial ligament (*1*) and its attachments to the posterior colliculus and talus. (From Pankovich AM, Shivaram MS. Anatomical basis of variability in injuries of the medial malleolus and the deltoid ligament. I. Anatomical studies. Acta Orthop Scand 1979;50:220.)

medial and the lateral measurements were never greater than 3 mm. Measurements between the medial malleolus and the medial surface of the talus were frequently 2 – 5 mm wider than the superior clear space, particularly on stress roentgenograms. From this study, it was concluded that the difference in width between the medial and the lateral clear space at the talar ridges greater than 3 mm indicates a rupture of the deep deltoid ligaments.

It must be noted that, following fixation of the fibular fracture, in cases in which the deltoid ligament is not repaired, or in which the medial malleolus is fixed but leaves some laxity of the deltoid ligament, or after fixation of the anterior colliculus in a concurrent lesion, intraoperative roentgenograms may show widening of the medial clear space (Fig. 9.10*A*). In most instances, the cause is external rotation of the talus, which brings the narrower part of the talar body forward and gives impression of widening. Holding the foot internally rotated, when applying the cast, will reduce the talus and show a normal mortise width on the roentgenogram (Fig. 9.10*B*).

Avulsion fractures of the posterior tubercle of the tibia by the posterior tibiofibular ligament are small fragments that do not contribute to instability of the ankle if the medial and lateral structures are repaired. Fixation of these small fragments is never necessary in my view. Larger fragments contribute significantly to instability of the ankle and must be fixed in an anatomic position. This type of fracture usually extends through the posterior process of the tibia and is produced by an axial compression force and represents a type of pilon fracture.

The last step in fixation of an ankle fracture is checking stability of the fibula in the fibular groove to assess injury to syndesmosis. Slight motion of 2–3 mm is

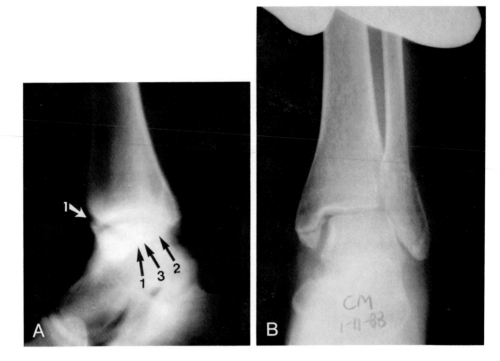

**Figure 9.5.** An isolated fracture of the anterior colliculus with an intact deep deltoid ligament attached to the posterior colliculus. **A**, Tomogram of the medial malleolus shows the fracture of the anterior colliculus (*1*), the intact posterior colliculus (*2*), and the intercollicular groove (*3*). **B**, A stress roentgenogram showed talar displacement of 2.5 mm, which indicated that the deep deltoid ligament was intact. The injury was treated with a short leg cast.

considered normal, whereas more significant motion requires insertion of a syndesmotic screw. I find the need for insertion of a syndesmotic screw exceedingly rare, perhaps once in 20–30 fractures. The screw should be removed 8 weeks later, since there is evidence (J Stiehl, personal communication) that leaving it in place may contribute to local discomfort, abnormal ankle motion, and possible screw fracture.

It is not quite clear what keeps the fibula stable in the syndesmosis after it has been fixed in an anatomic position. In some cases, it appears to be fixation of the medial malleolus, and yet failing to repair the deltoid ligament does not cause more instability. Danis-Weber classification offers some possible explanations for postfixation fibular stability, and there is some clinical and experimental evidence to confirm it (16). In type C, there are four subtypes characterized mainly by the extent of rupture of the interosseous membrane. In types C-1 and C-2, the interosseous membrane is ruptured to the level of the fracture, which is in the distal fibula. After fixation of these fractures, the stable proximal fibular fragment, attached to the intact interosseous membrane, provides stability to the entire fibula and to the syndesmosis. In types C-3 and C-4, the interosseous membrane is ruptured above the fracture site. Fixation of the fracture may not be sufficient to stabilize the entire fibula, thus the need for a syndesmotic screw.

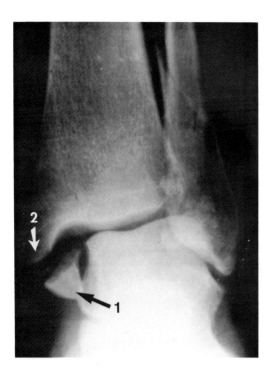

**Figure 9.6.** Concurrent fracture of the anterior colliculus and rupture of the deep deltoid ligament. Note displacement of the anterior colliculus (*1*), an intact posterior colliculus (*2*), and obviously wide displacement of the talus.

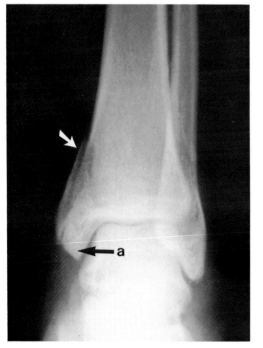

**Figure 9.7.** A fracture of the posterior colliculus. Note a typical supramalleolar spike (*arrow*) and an intact anterior colliculus (*a*).

**Figure 9.8.** The fractured posterior colliculus is best demonstrated on a roentgenogram taken with the ankle positioned in 20° of external rotation. *a*, Anterior colliculus. *b*, posterior colliculus.

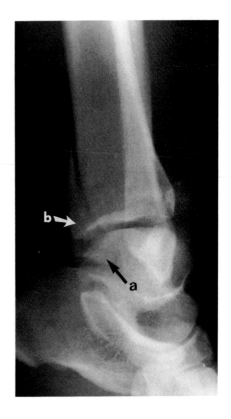

## AREAS FOR FUTURE CLINICAL INVESTIGATIONS

It is clear from the preceding presentation of ankle injuries that a number of problems in our understanding exist and need further investigation. It appears that topographic and functional anatomy of the deltoid ligament and medial malleolus has not been definitively settled, as new descriptions continue to appear in the literature. My view of this complex is that it is effectively divided into two parts. The anterior part consists of the anterior colliculus, to which the superficial deltoid ligaments are attached. The posterior part consists of the intercollicular groove and posterior colliculus, to which the deep deltoid (tibiotalar) ligament is attached. Clinical correlation demonstrated the following lesions: (*a*) fractures of the anterior and posterior colliculi, (*b*) concurrent fracture of the anterior colliculus and rupture of the deep deltoid ligament, (*c*) classical (supracollicular) fracture of the medial malleolus, and (*d*) rupture of the (entire) deltoid ligament. More recently, Rasmussen (15) described a different view of the deltoid ligament in which the anterior and the posterior parts (anterior and posterior tibiotalar) are considered a part of the deep portion and the middle part (tibiocalcaneal ligament) is the superficial portion. He also investigated multidirectional forces and consequent instabilities associated with ruptures of different portions of the deltoid ligament. However, it appeared that he did not consider lateral talar displacement, most important in determining stability in an ankle injury. Further work is clearly needed in this area.

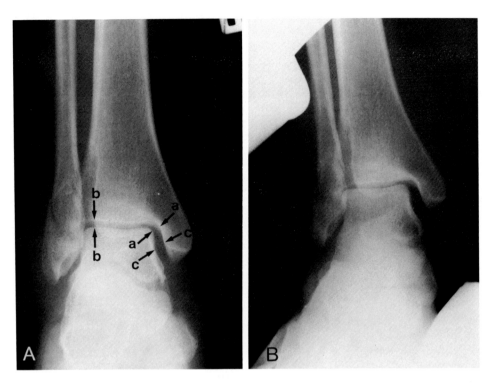

**Figure 9.9.**    Measurement of talar displacement as a test of rupture of the deep deltoid ligament. **A**, Measurements of the clear space are best taken at the medial and lateral sides of the plafond (*arrows aa* and *bb*). Space between the talus and the medial malleolus (*arrows cc*) is greater. **B**, External rotation stress roentgenogram. The talus has shifted at least 3 mm, indicating rupture of the deep deltoid ligament.

More investigation is needed to determine the mechanism of injury of various types of fibular fractures. There is recent evidence that plantar flexion or dorsiflexion of the foot may be as important as pronation/supination or rotation. Furthermore, as clinical patterns are observed, bone density, gender, and age of the patient seem to influence the type of fractures that are seen. The use of a syndesmotic screw continues to be controversial both in terms of when it is to be employed and for how long. It is not clear what keeps the fibula reduced after fixation of its fracture.

Finally, there is no good rationale to postoperative management. Is early postoperative motion necessary? What is the appropriate time to initiate weight bearing? My own impression is that most postoperative stiffness occurs in the subtalar joint and not the ankle joint. For that reason, I immobilize most patients for 5–6 weeks from the outset and expect to gain return of ankle motion in most cases. In patients with complete rupture of the deltoid ligament, I believe that 6 weeks of immobilization is mandatory.

In regard to early weight bearing, I studied a group of 20 young patients who had bimalleolar fractures fixed anatomically using the AO technique and for whom

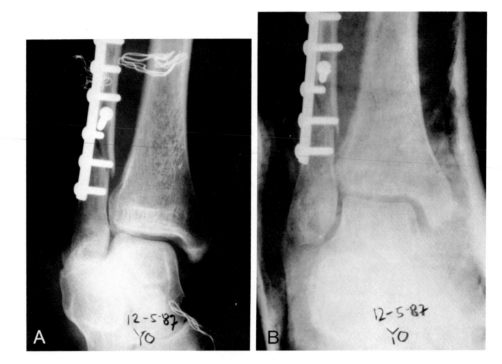

**Figure 9.10.** External rotational displacement of the talus indicates rupture or laxity of the deep deltoid ligament. **A,** An intraoperative roentgenogram showed significant displacement of the talus, due to its rotation, and consequent widening of the medial clear space. **B,** When the cast was being applied, the foot was internally rotated, thus closing the medial clear space and placing in proximity the ends of the ruptured deep deltoid ligament.

I advised early full weight bearing without a cast. Most of the patients had enough pain to avoid weight bearing for at least 4 weeks. From this study, I concluded that walking-cast immobilization for 5–6 weeks was more appropriate, and I continue to use it for most of my patients. However, more clinical experience is needed.

### References

1. Ashhurst APC, Bromer RC. Classification and mechanism of fractures of the long bones involving the ankle. Arch Surg 1922;4:51–129.
2. Bonnin JG. Injuries to the ankle. London: Heinemann Medical Books, Ltd, 1950.
3. Bosworth DM. Fracture-dislocation of the ankle with fixed displacement of the fibula behind the tibia. J Bone Joint Surg 1947;29;130–135.
4. Brostrom L. Sprained ankles. I. Anatomic lesions in recent sprains. Acta Chir Scand 1964;128:483–495.
5. Cedell C-A. Rupture of the posterior talotibial ligament with avulsion of a bone fragment from talus. Acta Orthop Scand 1974;45:454–461.
6. Close JR. Some applications of the functional anatomy of the ankle joint. J Bone Joint Surg 1956;38A:761–781.
7. Honigschmied J. Leichen experimente uber die Zerrissungen der Bander im Sprunggelenk, mit Rucksicht auf die Entstehung der indirecten Knockelfracturen. Deutsch Zschr Chir 1887;8:239–260.
8. Inman VT. The joints of the ankle. Baltimore: Williams & Wilkins, 1976.
9. Lauge-Hansen N. Fractures of the ankle. II. Combined experimental-surgical and experimental-roentgenologic investigations. Arch Surg 1950;60:957–985.

10. Lindstrand A. Lateral lesions in sprained ankles [Dissertation]. Lund, 1976.
11. Pankovich AM. Fractures of the fibula proximal to the distal tibio-fibular syndesmosis. J Bone Joint Surg 1978;60A:221–229.
12. Pankovich AM. Fractures of the fibula at the distal tibiofibular syndesmosis. Clin Orthop Relat Res 1979;143:138–147.
13. Pankovich AM, Shivaram MS. Anatomical basis of variability in injuries of the medial malleolus and the deltoid ligament. I. Anatomical studies. Acta Orthop Scand 1979;50:217–223.
14. Pankovich AM, Shivaram MS. Anatomical basis of variability in injuries of the medial malleolus and the deltoid ligament. II. Clinical studies. Acta Orthop Scand 1979;50:225–236.
15. Rasmussen O. Stability of the ankle joint: Analysis of the function and traumatology of the ankle ligaments. Acta Orthop Scand Suppl 1985;211:56.
16. Riegels-Nielsen P, Christensen J, Greiff J. The stability of tibiofibular syndesmosis following rigid internal fixation for type C malleolar fractures: An experimental and clinical study. Injury 1983;14:357–360.
17. Wagstaffe WW. An unusual form of fracture of the fibula. St Thomas Hosp Rep 1875;6:43–47.

# Appendices

## INTRODUCTION

Inman studied the morphology and simple kinematic relationships of the ankle and subtalar joints using ingenious but rather simple devices. Most studies were performed on embalmed cadaver specimens supplemented with freshly amputated specimens. Inman discounted the effect of embalming on the articular cartilage and removed all soft tissues from joints where motion was studied. Furthermore, he found through experience that a constant force between 4.5 and 9 kg on each joint was optimal to obtain reproducible joint measurements.

The designs of joint articulators and descriptions of other accessory apparatuses is beyond the scope of this section. However, the editor felt that this information is paramount to understanding the various studies performed by Inman. Pictures of all devices and techniques will be published as represented in the original edition. It is hoped that the reader will find this section stimulating and relevant.

## Appendix A

# Method of locating the ankle axis and obtaining various measurements

**Step 1.** The tibia is fixed firmly in the clamp of the articulator. The fibula remains free so that lateral or rotatory displacements of this bone can be detected during movement of the joint (Fig. A-1).

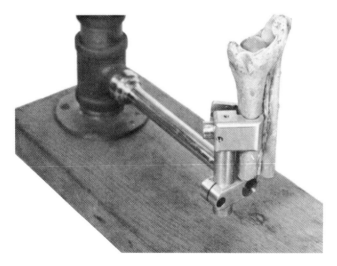

**Figure A-1.** Tibia held rigidly in clamp on articulator, with fibula free so that any movement can be detected.

**Step 2.** The disarticulated talus is fixed in its holder (Fig. A-2).

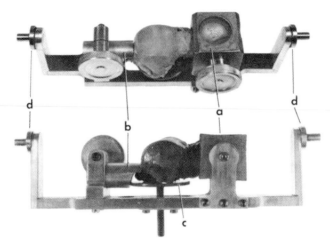

**Figure A-2.**   Holder for talus. *a*, Rotating block with hemispherical concavities of four different dimensions for reception of head of talus, which varies in size; *b*, adjustable tube provided with lip to fix nonarticular posterior ledge of talus; *c*, movable platform to provide three-point fixation of talus; *d*, arms supporting pins for attachment to articulator. The centers of the pins are on approximately the same level as the surface of the trochlea. This ensures stability of the holder when placed in the articulator and also permits the holder to swivel freely and maintain lateral contact between the articular surfaces.

**Step 3.** The talus in its holder is inverted and articulated within the ankle mortise (Fig. A-3).

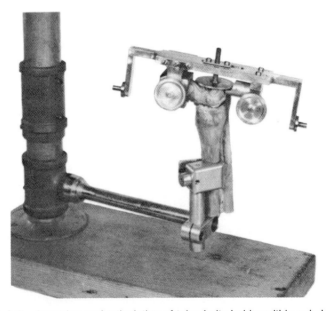

**Figure A-3.**   Inversion and articulation of talus in its holder within ankel mortise.

**Step 4.** The articulator, supporting the talus in its mortise, is assembled. Accuracy of fit and smoothness of motion are checked while the joint is carried through its full range of motion (Fig. A-4).

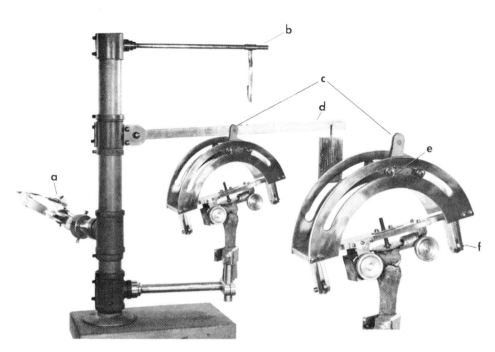

**Figure A-4.** Completely assembled articulator. *a*, Axis locator carrying pointers in a stirrup, swung away for initial assembly of articulator. *b*, Arm with hook to support lever arm with 4.5-kg weight and articulator while talus in its holder is being placed in mortise. *c*, Short linkage placed between lever arm and remainder of articulator. This linkage permits 2 cm of horizontal travel and transmits 9 kg of force perpendicular to the articulating surfaces of the bones during movement of the talus in its mortise. *d*, Lever arm, acting as compression bar, supporting 4.5-kg weight. *e*, Carriage, traveling on double circular track, permitting rotation of talus in its mortise. A bearing placed between the short linkage and the carriage allows free rotation of the carriage in a horizontal plane. *f*, Slotted bars to receive pins on talus holder, allowing it to swivel within mortise.

**Step 5.** The adjustable axis locator is manipulated until the pointers are directed toward the points on the medial and lateral sides of the talus, which demonstrate minimal displacement as the talus is rotated in the articulator from full flexion to full extension. The pointer on one side is located, then pressed into the cortex of the bone to fix it firmly. The axis locator is manipulated on the opposite side of the bone until its pointer is over a point of minimal motion. It is also pushed into the cortex. This determines an external axis (two pointers) about which the talus must move. The accuracy of the location of the axis is now checked by rotating the talus and observing the degree of contact between the articulating surfaces of the joint (Fig. A-5).

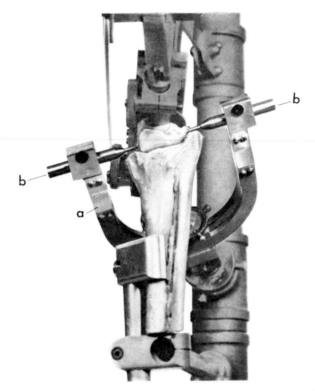

**Figure A-5.**   End view of carriage, with axis locator in place. *a*, Stirrup, adjustable in all directions and carrying sharpened pointers. *b*, Pointers carried on 10-mm stainless steel rods to assure rigidity.

**Step 6.**  All adjustments on the axis locator are rigidly fixed.

**Step 7.**  Motion of the talus in its mortise is again checked to confirm the accuracy of the positioning pointers.

**Step 8.** The pointers are removed from the stirrup of the axis locator and replaced with drill guides, and a 3-mm hole is drilled through the talus (Fig. A-6).

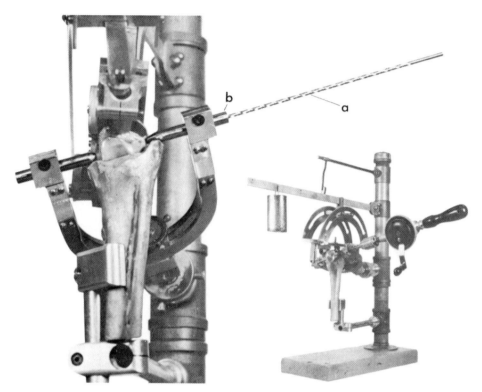

**Figure A-6.** Establishment of rigid axis. *a*, 3-mm stainless steel drill; *b*, hollow drill guides. The *smaller figure* shows drilling of the hole through the talus controlled by the hollow drill guides that replaced the pointers in the axis locator stirrup.

**Step 9.** The drill is removed and replaced with a stainless steel rod (15 cm in length and 3 mm in diameter). The talus is disengaged from its holder, and the upper portion of the articulator, with its 9 kg of force, is removed. The movement of the talus in the mortise is checked for maximal contact of the articular surfaces and smoothness of movement; the talus is now forced to rotate around the fixed axis determined by the 3-mm stainless steel rod held rigidly in its stirrup (Fig. A-7).

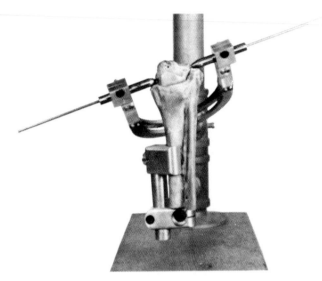

**Figure A-7.** Apparatus with articulator and talus holder removed. The talus remains rigidly fixed by the 3-mm stainless steel rod held in the axis locator. Movement of the talus within the mortise is checked as it is forced to rotate about a fixed axis.

**Step 10.** The measurement of the angle between the plafond of the mortise and the midline of the tibia required the use of a special goniometer. The plafond is concave in an anteroposterior plane and it has a slight medial elevation. To determine a plane that would closely correspond to the average inclination of the plafond, two hemidisks fixed to a movable slide were added to the goniometer. The isolated goniometer is shown in Figure A-8 and its application is shown in Figure A-9. Without loosening the axis locator with the drill guides, the stainless steel pin is withdrawn and the talus is removed from the mortise. The angle between the surface of the mortise (plafond) and the center line of the tibia is measured with the goniometer (Fig. A-10).

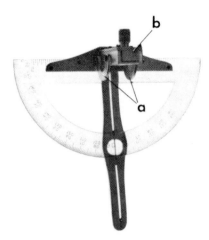

**Figure A-8.** Posterior view of special goniometer. *a*, Two hemidisks fixed to movable slide. These orient the edge of the protractor to a plane which corresponds to the lateral and medial articular surfaces and ignores the variable medial elevation. *b*, Movable slide permitting hemidisks to be adjusted so as to contact bottom of anteroposterior concavity of plafond.

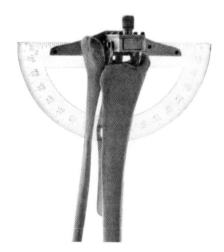

**Figure A-9.** Posterior view of goniometer applied to dry bony specimen to demonstrate positioning of hemidisks within mortise.

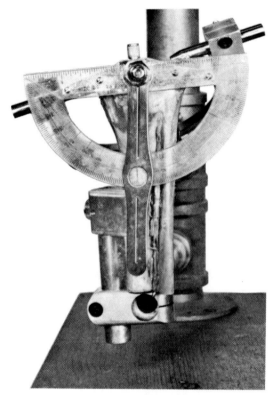

**Figure A-10.**   Use of special goniometer to determine angle between plafond of mortise and long axis of tibia.

**Step 11.** The angle between the empirically determined axis through the talus and the center line of the tibia is measured with a second goniometer that has curved brackets that fit over the drill guides so that it aligns itself parallel to the axis (Fig. A-11).

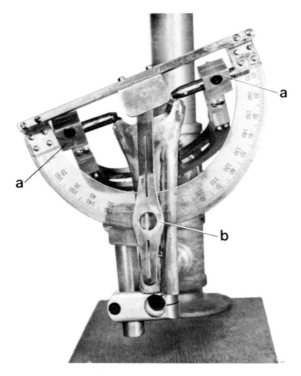

**Figure A-11.** Second goniometer constructed to determine angle between empirically located axis of ankle joint and midline of tibia. *a*, Shallow stirrups located at each end of frames supporting protractor and fitting over drill guides, which correspond to empirical axis. *b*, Movable arm for measuring angle between axis and midline of tibia.

**Step 12.** The stainless steel rod (without the talus) is reinserted through the guide holes in the axis locator stirrup. Masking tape is wrapped around the periphery of the mortise and extended upward to include the stainless steel rod representing the empirically determined axis of the ankle joint. The receptacle formed by the mortise and its surrounding masking tape is filled with liquid dental stone to a height sufficient to enclose the stainless steel rod. The preparation is tapped gently to cause the dental stone to fill all crevices (Fig. A-12).

**Step 13.** After the dental stone has set, it is removed; it provides an accurate mold of the mortise and includes the empirically determined ankle axis. This cast is labeled and set aside for further study.

**Step 14.** The tibia with the fibula and the talus are removed from the clamp and replaced in preserving fluid to prevent drying while awaiting further study.

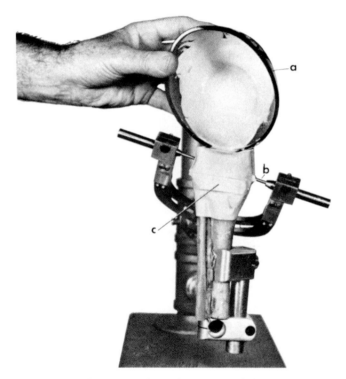

**Figure A-12.** Method for taking cast of mortise. *a,* Liquid dental stone; *b,* 3-mm axis rod reinserted through drill guides to relate empirical axis to cast; *c,* receptacle of masking tape to contain dental stone.

# Appendix B

# Methods used for the measurement
# of trochlear widths

**Method (According to Barnett and Napier, 1952) Employed to Measure the Widths of the Trochleas in Planes Always Perpendicular to the Surfaces of the Tibial Facets.** A small flat stainless steel plate was rigidly fixed to one arm of a compass, in a plane at a right angle to the plane of the compass. On the other arm of the compass was an adjustable pointer (Fig. B-1). This special caliper was constructed and used in the following manner.

The flat plate was held firmly against the surface of the tibial facet and the calipers were closed until the pointer contacted the lateral (fibular) surface of the trochlea (Fig. B-2). Since the edge joining the superior surface of the trochlea and the fibular facet was always rounded, it was necessary to place the tip of the pointer on the spot that appeared to represent the superior border of the true surface of the fibular facet.

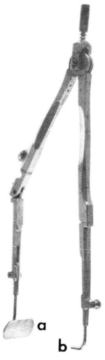

**Figure B-1.** Calipers employed to measure width of trochlea at right angle to plane of tibial facet. *a*, Flat plate for surface of tibial facet; *b*, blunt pointer for fibular facet.

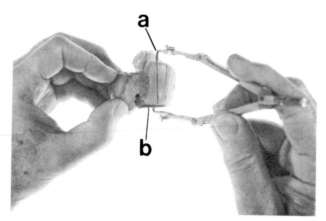

**Figure B-2.** Method of employing calipers to measure width of trochlea. *a*, Pointer applied to fibular facet; *b*, flat plate applied to tibial facet.

When the posterior width of the trochlea was measured, the flattened triangular facet (for the inferior transverse ligament of the tibiofibular syndesmosis) was included in the width. Three dimensions were measured, one at the anterior margin, one in the approximate center, and the last at the posterior margin of the articular surface of the fibular facet. Measurements were made to the nearest millimeter and recorded. Cadaver specimens (107) were used.

    **Method Employed to Measure the Widths of the Trochleas and Their Mortises along "Saw Cuts."** Specimens used in this study consisted of tali and the casts of their corresponding mortises, in which saw cuts had been made (see Appendix E). The length of each saw cut in the trochleas (Fig. B-3) and their corresponding casts (Fig. B-4) was measured with a pair of bow dividers. The arms of the dividers were fitted with extensions of 2-mm stainless steel rods bent and provided with small tapered nibs. The nibs held the pointers in the ends of the saw cuts as the dividers were closed to contact the articular surfaces. The measurements were taken at the superior margins of the true tibial and fibular facets. The dimensions were recorded to the nearest millimeter in 107 tali and casts of mortises. The beveled triangular area of the posterolateral aspect of the trochlea was included in the measured width.

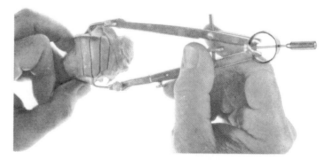

**Figure B-3.** Bow dividers being used to measure width of trochlea along saw cuts in talus.

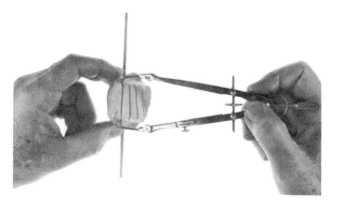

**Figure B-4.** Bow dividers being used to measure width of mortise along saw cuts in cast of mortise.

# Appendix C

## Method used to measure the angles between the vertical planes of the fibular and tibial facets and the empirically located axis of the ankle joint

A special goniometer was constructed. It consisted of a plastic protractor mounted on a movable mechanical parallelogram. One arm of the mechanical parallelogram was rigidly fixed parallel to a 3-mm stainless steel rod. The longer arm of the rod was for insertion into the drill hole previously made (see Appendix A), which represented the ankle axis. The shorter arm carried a pointer. The scale was free to move with one arm of the parallelogram (Fig. C-1).

The rod was inserted through the drill hole, and the angles between the ankle axis and the tibial facet (Fig. C-2*A*) and the ankle axis and the fibular facet (Fig. C-2*B*) were measured. The surfaces of the tibial facets were reasonably flat. The fibular facets were curved to varying extents, requiring that a tangent be estimated by eye. The accuracy of the angular measurements on the fibular side, therefore, was

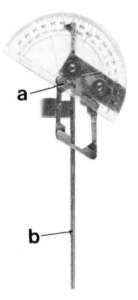

**Figure C-1.** Goniometer for measuring angle between planes of tibial and fibular facets and empirically located axis of ankle joint. *a*, Movable protractor attached to one side of parallelogram; *b*, rod for insertion into drill hole in talus, which orients goniometer to ankle axis.

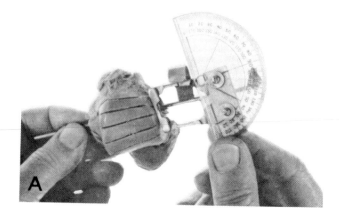

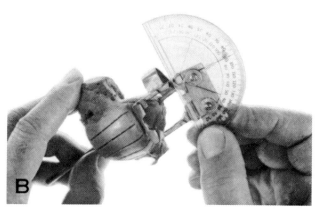

**Figure C-2.**   Method of measuring angles between planes of tibial and fibular facets and axis of ankle joint. **A**, Tibial facet; **B**, fibular facet.

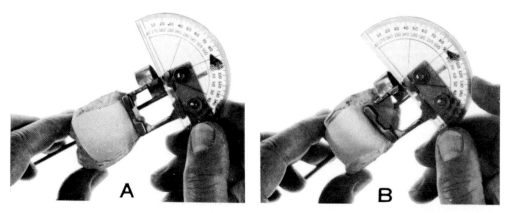

**Figure C-3.**   Method of measuring angles of tibial (**A**) and fibular (**B**) facets on casts of mortises.

not as precise as one would desire. However, repeated measurements upon the same specimen on different days and by different investigators showed the individual measurements to be within 4° of one another.

The casts of the mortises were measured in a manner similar to that used for the tali (Fig. C-3). A series of 107 cadaver tali and casts were measured in this manner. The results are given in the text.

# Appendix D

## Methods used to determine the curvatures of the superior surfaces of the trochleas and their corresponding casts

In this study of the curvature of the trochlea, three procedures and several different pieces of equipment were employed. In all 107 specimens, the contourometer was used. In 59 specimens, the "Formagage" was employed as a rapid check, and in a selected group of 30 specimens, a visual check was added in which a modified caliper was used.

It is apparent that, in studying a convex surface, all three of the techniques are readily applicable. However, in measuring the curvature of a concave surface, neither the contourometer nor the caliper could be satisfactorily used, since the data would consist in estimating the movement of a point. Therefore, casts of the mortises (see Appendix A) were employed and measured precisely, as were the tali.

**The Contourometer.** A special apparatus was constructed (Fig. D-1). It consisted of two metal turntables mounted on ball bearings and connected by gears and a chain. No play occurred between the turntables. In the center of one was a shaft into which a 3-mm rod could be inserted and fixed with a thumbscrew. Each talus (or cast) with its 3-mm rod representing the empirically located axis of the ankle joint (see Appendix A) was securely held to its metal axis by two collars with projecting prongs. The axial rod was mounted in the shaft of the turntable. The talus or cast could then be rotated in space about its empirically determined axis. Firmly fixed to the base of the apparatus was a vertical member that carried a movable horizontal arm. At one end of the arm was an adjustable rod carrying a tiny ball bearing (3 mm). The outer race of the bearing contacted the articular surface of the trochlea, providing smooth and relatively frictionless movement.

At the other end of the movable horizontal arm was mounted a spring-loaded ball-point pen, which played against the surface of the second turntable. A card (10 × 15 cm) could be placed on the surface of the turntable and held with four microscope slide clips. The apparatus was tested for accuracy of reproduction using various irregularly shaped sections of plastic rods (see Fig. D-1).

After the specimens were mounted, they were rotated through an angular range permitted by the articular surfaces. Three contours were recorded, one at the most lateral edge, one at the medial edge, and one in the approximate center. The position of each contour was marked on each talus with an indelible pencil and transferred to the cast of its corresponding mortise. This was necessary for making comparable measurements between the cadaver tali and their casts.

The data reduction was similar to that used with the Formagage and will be described below.

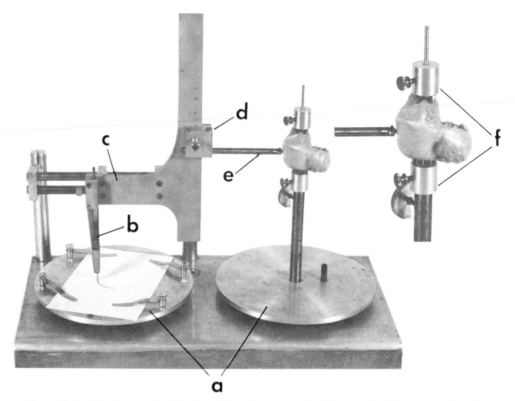

**Figure D-1.** Contourometer. The *inset* shows in greater detail the method of mounting the talus (or the cast of the mortise) on the axle of one turntable and the small (3-mm) ball bearing, which contacted the articular surface of the trochlea. *a*, Turntables linked together by gears and a bicycle chain within base of contourometer. *b*, Spring-loaded ball-point pen for recording curvature on data card. *c*, Horizontal slide for transmission of displacement of contour rod to ball-point pen. Constant contact of the contour rod with its ball bearing was maintained by rubber bands not visible in the photograph. *d*, Vertical slide for adjusting contour rod to desired levels on trochlea. *e*, Contour rod carrying small ball bearing. *f*, Collars for holding talus.

**The Formagage.** The Formagage is an instrument for contouring irregular surfaces. Its use is simple and convenient and is clearly depicted in Figure D-2. When used, it was held as nearly perpendicular as possible to the 3-mm rod representing the ankle axis. After contouring of the surface of the specimen, the instrument was locked and the curvature was transferred with a sharply pointed pencil to the data cards (Fig. D-2).

The curvature of each specimen was recorded on cards with information derived from either the contourometer or the Formagage. A transparent plastic overlay was precision-engraved with circles of varying radii with 2-mm increments. The recorded arcs were matched as accurately as possible to the inscribed circles in the plastic overlay (Fig. D-3), in order to locate the arc and its center. At this center a circle was drawn with a compass; then the extent to which the recorded curvature deviated from the arc of a true circle could be readily determined.

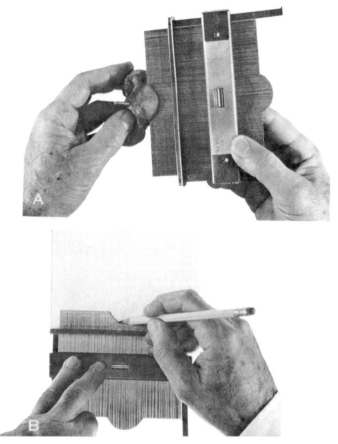

**Figure D-2.** Formagage. **A**, Method of using Formagage to obtain curvature of trochlea; **B**, transference of curvature to data card after gage is locked.

In the complete series of 107 tali, 86 of the recorded curvatures could be fitted to an arc of a circle within 1 mm. Reproductions of typical data cards are shown in Figure D-4. In the remaining 21 tali, one or more of the recorded contour curves could not be accurately fitted to an arc of a circle. An example of one of the poorest fits is shown in Figure D-4 (*lower card*).

It was thought that the inability to demonstrate the curvature of the trochlea of the talus to be an arc of a true circle in 20% (21/107) of the specimens might be due to errors in the two techniques employed. Therefore, these 21 specimens and selected specimens showing good circularity were rechecked with a specially modified pair of calipers; a 3-mm rod was inserted into one arm and an adjustable pointer into the other. The rod was inserted into the drill hole of the specimen and the dividers were closed until the pointer contacted the articular surface of the trochlea (Fig. D-5). The caliper was rotated and deviations from circularity could be readily seen. This visual check confirmed the accuracy of both the contourometer and the Formagage and demonstrated the noncircularity of the 21 specimens. A review of the data showed

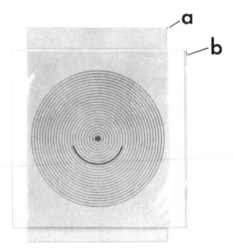

**Figure D-3.** Method of determining center of arc of curvature of trochlea obtained from contourometer or Formagage. *a*, Data card on which arc of curvature has been recorded; *b*, precision-engraved plastic overlay used to determine center of recorded arcs.

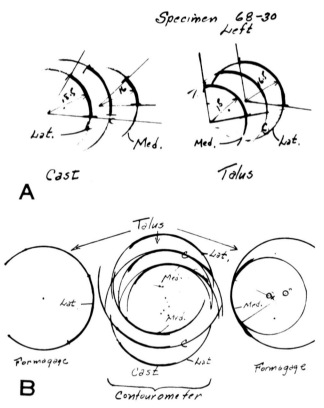

**Figure D-4.** Samples of typical data cards. With use of the centers determined from the plastic overlay, arcs of circles have been drawn with a compass. Coincidence or deviations of the contours from true circularity can be readily seen. The *upper card* shows good coincidence while the *lower card* shows deviations.

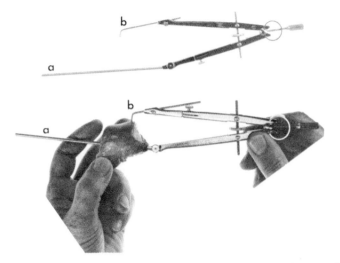

**Figure D-5.** Modified calipers used to visually check circularity of trochlear surface. *a*, 3-mm rod for insertion into hole representing previously determined empirical axis. *b*, Adjustable pointer to contact articular surface of trochlea as caliper is rotated around its fixed axis running through talus.

that deviations from arcs of circles occurred almost exclusively on the medial side. Nineteen specimens, while demonstrating circularity on the lateral side of the trochlea, deviated from circularity on the medial side. Two specimens demonstrated noncircularity on both sides.

The data cards of the 86 tali, which demonstrated good circularity of the trochlea, were selected for measurement of the radii of curvature. The radii were measured from the circles inscribed on the cards and represented the medial and lateral sides. The radius of the middle contour was not measured. The arcs of circles for the casts were also available on the same data card, having been contoured at the same relative locations as their tali (Fig. D-4). Measurements were made to the nearest half-millimeter on a steel scale.

The data were tabulated and comparisons were made between the radii on the two sides of the talus and between corresponding radii on the talus and the cast of the mortise.

# Appendix E

## Method employed to visually demonstrate the conical shape of the trochlea by means of saw cuts

The use of saw cuts into the trochlea to demonstrate that they converged toward the medial side was first made on a freshly amputated undissected ankle by Close and Inman (1952). This procedure was modified and extended in an anthropometric study of 107 cadaver specimens. Several pieces of equipment were constructed to expedite the making of the saw cuts and to measure the conical angle on each talus and on the cast of its corresponding mortise.

**Saw Guide (Fig. E-1).** A 9-mm metallic bow was constructed, which could be rotated in two planes and locked to a heavy plastic (Formica) plate. At both ends of the bow were 3-mm holes with setscrews to receive and fix the 3-mm rod representing the empirical axis of the ankle joint. Immediately above the 3-mm screw holes were slotted extensions for the blade of a hack saw. The slots were aligned so that the saw blade lay in the same vertical plane as the 3-mm rod representing the empirical axis of the ankle joint. A circular arm was attached at a right angle to the center of the bow, on which graduation marks were imprinted at 15° intervals. Through a chuck, mounted on this arm, a threaded screw pin could be inserted into the talus or the cast for fixation and graduated motion.

In use, the talus (or cast) was placed in the center of the bow. A 15-cm rod, 3 mm in diameter, was inserted through the bow and the drill hole in the talus. The specimen was fixed by the threaded pin. The talus was rotated until either the posterior or anterior edge of the articular surface of the trochlea lay in the vertical plane of the saw blade. All movable parts were rigidly fixed with thumbscrews. With a saw, a cut approximately 6 mm deep was made into the trochlea. The saw blade was elevated and the talus was rotated 15° about its empirical axis. The specimen was again rigidly clamped and another saw cut was made. This procedure was repeated until saw cuts had been made over the entire trochlear surface. Usually, there were four to six cuts per specimen (Fig. E-2). In no specimens were the saw cuts parallel; they converged toward the medial side of the talus or cast.

**Measurement of the Conical Angle.** To determine the angle of convergence of the saw cuts and to calculate the average conical angle of each trochlea and cast, a special goniometer was constructed (Fig. E-3). This consisted of a wooden base 51 cm long, provided with two 7.6-cm brass pillars 46 cm apart. A 3-mm rod passed through holes in each pillar and supported the talus by passing through the drill hole of the ankle axis. A 1-mm stainless steel pin was forcibly pushed into one of the saw cuts. Because the center of the trochlea exhibited a slight concavity of varying depth, the pin was made flush with the medial and lateral surfaces only and the central

125

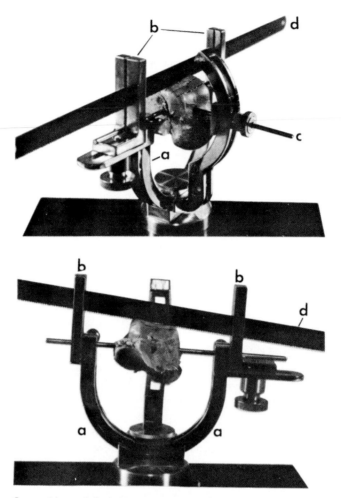

**Figure E-1.** Saw guide. *a*, Adjustable metal bow supporting talus on 3-mm rod that represents empirical axis; *b*, slotted saw guides; *c*, screw pin inserted into nonarticular part of talus and held in chuck, which can be moved along circular track to turn and fix talus in various degrees of rotation; *d*, saw blade from which frame has been removed.

concavity was ignored. The talus was rotated until the pin in the saw cut lay in the same horizontal plane as the rod representing the ankle axis. In most of the specimens, the saw cut pin crossed this rod at varying distances and angles on the medial side of the specimen.

A plastic protractor was mounted horizontally in such a way that it could be slid toward or away from the specimen until the center of the protractor overlay the point of intersection of the axis rod and the pin in the saw cuts. The angle between rod and pin was recorded to the nearest estimated degree.

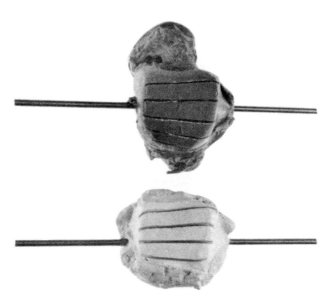

**Figure E-2.**   Typical talus and cast of its mortise after saw cuts have been made.

The procedure was repeated for each saw cut. Because of various factors, the differences between individual measurements on each saw cut differed from 1 to 5°, so that there were inaccuracies of this magnitude inherent in the method. In the hope that the variations were randomly distributed, the four to six measurements were averaged for each specimen.

The conical angle of the trochlea was calculated for each specimen by multiplying the average angle of convergence of the saw cuts by two.

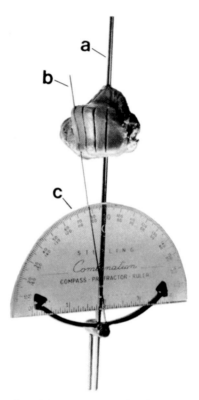

**Figure E-3.** Goniometer employed to measure angle of convergence of saw cuts. *a*, 3-mm stainless steel rod on which talus and protractor are mounted; *b*, stiff stainless steel Kirschner wire pressed into saw cut; *c*, protractor, which is slid along axis rod until its center lies over point of intersection of Kirschner wire and 3-mm axis rod.

# Appendix F

## Method of locating the subtalar axis, measuring the range of motion about it, and analyzing the "screwlike" motion of the talus on the calcaneus

**Location of the Subtalar Axis (Fig. F-1).** The calcaneus is firmly held in a clamp (Fig. F-1, *a*) rigidly fixed to a pipe frame.

The talus is articulated on the calcaneus. Sharp pointers (as employed in Appendix A) are inserted into the stirrup (Fig. F-1, *b*). The stirrup is moved by means of a jointed support until the talar pointer locates the point of minimal motion on the talus as it is moved through its full range while the articular surfaces are manually held in contact. The talar pointer is driven into the bone sufficiently to mark the point of minimal motion. The process is then reversed, the talus is clamped, and the calcaneus is moved on the talus. The point of minimal motion on the calcaneus is

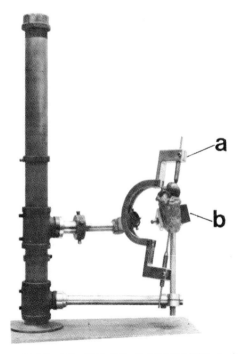

**Figure F-1.** Apparatus used to determine axis of subtalar joint. *a*, Adjustable stirrup holding same pointers and drill guides as were employed for studies described in Appendix A; *b*, clamp to secure calcaneus (or talus).

located. The stirrup is adjusted until the two pointers, when gently pressed into the bone, align the two points of minimal motion. Accuracy of location of the functional axis is checked by moving the joint through its range of motion and observing any restriction of motion or movement of the pointers, as well as preservation of contact of the articular surfaces.

The stirrup is locked and the pointers are replaced with drill guides. The stirrup now acts as a jig for the drill. A 3-mm drill is passed through both bones and replaced with a 3-mm stainless steel rod (see Fig. F-1). The two bones are removed from the apparatus and the accuracy of placement of the axis is checked. If restriction of motion or separation of articular surfaces has occurred, the process of axis location is repeated.

All tali and calcanei were left articulated, with their 3-mm stainless steel axes in place, and returned to containers with preservative fluid until used for further study.

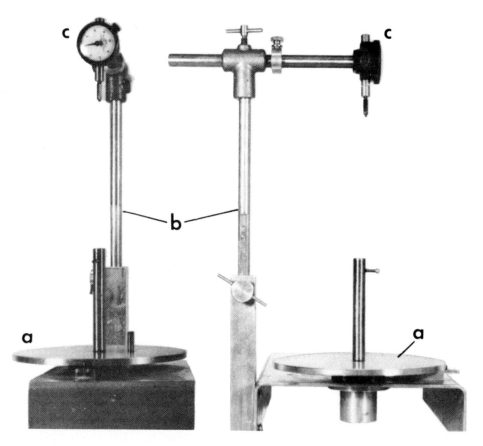

**Figure F-2.** Apparatus for studying alleged screwlike motion of talus on calcaneus. *a*, Calibrated turntable with axle drilled to accept 3-mm stainless steel rod; *b*, adjustable frame supporting dial gage; *c*, dial gage calibrated to 0.025 mm.

**Series I (47 Specimens).** Since only ranges of motion were being considered in this series, the method consisted of clamping the calcaneus and mounting a protractor perpendicular to the stainless steel rod, with constituted the functional axis. A flexible pointer was drilled into the fixed calcaneus. Rotation of the talus with its protractor revealed the range of motion.

Two sets of measurements were made on each specimen. The first set of measurements was made with capsular and ligamentous structures intact and the second, with all ligamentous restraints removed.

**Series II.** The intent of this study on cadaver tali and calcanei was to reinvestigate the screwlike motion of the talus on the calcaneus. Such action had been reported in the literature. Two separate series of measurements were made. The first consisted of an investigation of the curvature of the posterior facet of the calcaneus, in an attempt to collect data from which a helix angle could be calculated. The second was a series of direct measurements on the absolute linear displacement of the talus along its empirically determined axis during rotation of the talus on the calcaneus.

In both studies the basic apparatus consisted of a turntable with a protruding axle. The axle had been drilled to receive the 3-mm stainless steel rod. The turntable had been calibrated for rotation to $1°$. To an outrigger was fixed a dial gage calibrated to 0.025 mm (Fig. F-2).

For the studies of the curvature of the posterior facet of the calcaneus, the talus was removed and the calcaneus was rigidly mounted on the turntable. The arm carrying the dial gage was adjusted to contact the articular surface and to record deflections over the entire extent of the articular surface as the turntable rotated the calcaneus. The articular surface was contoured at 5 and 10 mm from the center of the empirical axis. Recordings from the dial gage were made for every $10°$ of rotation (Fig. F-3).

The curves of the plotted values showed such individual variations that it was felt of interest to present the actual data on 10 of the 49 specimens studied. These were selected as representative of typical patterns and are reproduced in Figures F-4 through F-7.

To measure the absolute linear displacement of the talus along the empirical axis, the turntable was locked and a protractor was fixed to the shaft to record rotations. The talus was articulated upon the calcaneus. The 3-mm rod representing the empirical axis was extended into the talus but only sufficiently far to assure that rotation of the talus occurred around it. The upper end of the rod was left approximately 5 mm short of protruding from the neck of the talus. To provide a flat surface perpendicular to the arm of the dial gage, a flat-headed copper rivet was gently pushed into the drill hole left unoccupied by the rod. The shank of the rivet was not long enough to contact the axial rod, and its fit in the drill hole was sufficiently snug to force it to follow all motions of the talus. To record the amount of rotation of the talus upon the fixed calcaneus, a pointer was inserted in the talus. The stem of the dial gage was lowered to contact the head of the rivet, the talus was rotated, and recordings from the dial gage for every $10°$ of rotation were made (Fig. F-8).

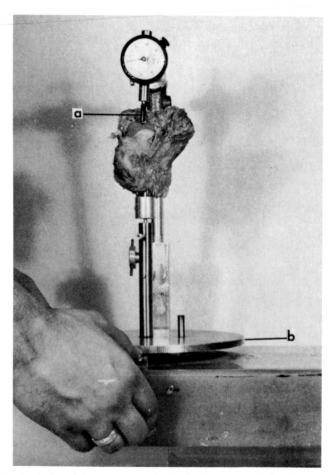

**Figure F-3.** Method of studying curvature of posterior facet of calcaneus. *a*, Stem of dial gage contacting articular surface of posterior facet of calcaneus at measured distance (5 or 10 mm) from center of axis; *b*, calibrated turntable. Recordings from the dial gage were made at every 10° of rotation of the turntable.

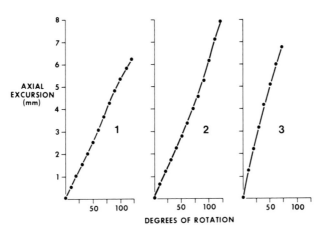

**Figure F-4.** Plotted data on three specimens, which are representative of a group constituting over half of specimens studied. Note that the loci may be fitted with a straight line and that although the slopes of the curves differ they suggest a pure screwlike behavior of the subtalar joint.

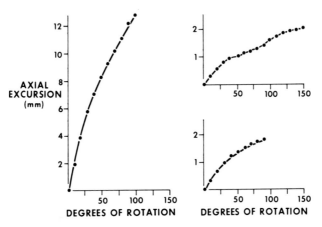

**Figure F-5.** Curves revealing progressive linear displacement. The increments are not constant, however, and therefore indicate that the joint is not behaving as a true screw.

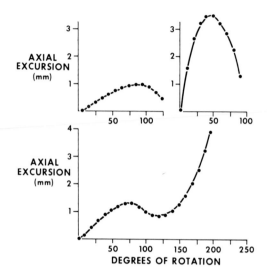

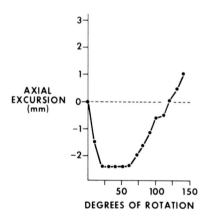

**Figure F-6.** Curves revealing reversal in linear displacements, indicating divergence from true screwlike behavior.

**Figure F-7.** Curve representing findings in nine specimens. The initial displacement is negative, indicating a left-handed screw. There is a reversal to a right-handed screw at the termination of rotation, resulting in a total linear displacement of only 1 mm.

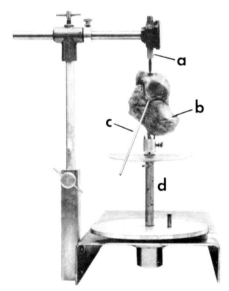

**Figure F-8.**   Apparatus to measure linear displacement of talus along axis of subtalar joint, with rotation of talus upon calcaneus. *a*, Stem of dial gage resting upon flat head of rivet that has been inserted into axis hole in talus; *b*, calcaneus rigidly fixed to axle of turntable; *c*, rod inserted into talus to rotate it upon fixed calcaneus, with amount of rotation indicated on protractor; *d*, turntable locked in position with protractor rigidly mounted on axle.

# Appendix G

## Method of determining the angles between the axis of the subtalar joint and the calcaneofibular ligament and between the anterior talofibular and calcaneofibular ligaments

In 50 cadaver specimens, all soft tissues were removed except the collateral ligaments of the ankle, which were carefully preserved. Most specimens were soaked in water for several days to make them more pliable. The subtalar axis was determined and a 3-mm stainless steel rod was inserted as outlined in Appendix F. A 1-mm Kirschner wire was threaded through the calcaneofibular ligament parallel to the direction of its fibers. A similar, but shorter, 1-mm Kirschner wire was inserted through the fibers of the anterior talofibular ligament and permitted to extend laterally (Fig. G-1).

**The Angle Between the Calcaneofibular Ligament and the Axis of the Subtalar Joint.** The tibia was firmly held in a clamp and fixed to a support stand by an adjustable holder. With a slight adjustment of the specimen, the rod and wire were made to lie in the same vertical plane (Fig. G-2). The angle between the two, as measured in this plane, was felt to represent the true angle of divergence between the rod and the wire.

To measure the angle between the rod and the wire a goniometer held in a horizontal plane on a separate stand was moved over the specimen and adjusted to measure the angle (Fig. G-3) in three positions of the subtalar joint: full inversion of the calcaneus, the approximate midposition, and full eversion of the calcaneus. The angular change between the rod and the wire was recorded in three positions in 50 specimens. In all specimens, in the midposition of the subtalar joint the direction of the fibers of the calcaneofibular ligament paralleled the axis of the subtalar joint surprisingly closely. The maximal deviation of about 10° from true parallelism in a few specimens could be due to errors in the location of the axis rod and in the insertion of the wire into the calcaneofibular ligament, failure to select the true midposition of the joint, and sloppy positioning of the goniometer. The average angle between the rod and the wire in the midposition of the subtalar joint was 0° ± 8°. When the leg and foot were visualized in the anatomic standing position, i.e., foot flat and leg vertical as customarily depicted in textbooks, a positive value of the angle indicated that the direction of the fibers of the calcaneofibular ligament was slightly more vertical than the axis of the subtalar joint. A negative value indicated that the fibers of the calcaneofibular ligament were slightly more horizontal than the axis of the subtalar joint. When the calcaneus was maximally inverted or everted around the subtalar axis, the degree of parallelism between the axis rod and the wire (representing the calcaneofibular ligament) was slightly decreased. With maximal inversion and

137

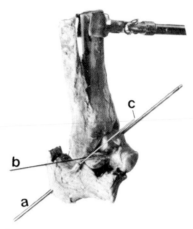

**Figure G-1.**   Oblique view of typical specimen. *a*, Rod inserted through talus and calcaneus in position of empirically located axis of subtalar joint; *b*, Kirschner wire inserted into anterior talofibular ligament paralleling its fibers; *c*, Kirschner wire inserted into calcaneofibular ligament paralleling its fibers.

eversion, the direction of the fibers deviated from true parallelism by a maximal value of 19° and a minimal value of 2°. The average deviation was 14° ± 9°. The differences in the extent of deviation from parallelism with inversion and eversion of the calcaneus seem to be due to variations, in individual specimens, between the location of the calcaneal attachment of the ligament and the position of the axis rod as it emerged on the lateral side of the calcaneus. In those specimens in which the calcaneal attachment was closest to the exit of the axis rod on the lateral side of the calcaneus, there was less deviation from parallelism with inversion and eversion of the calcaneus. In all specimens, however, the ligament in no way limited the full range of movement in the subtalar joint, and in no position was the ligament unduly taut or lax.

**The Angle as Projected onto the Transverse Plane.** When the positions of the rod representing the axis of the subtalar joint and the Kirschner wire through

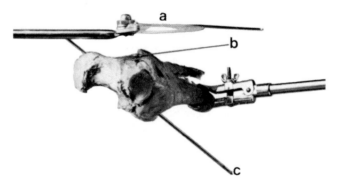

**Figure G-2.**   Specimen oriented so that axis rod and Kirschner wire in calcaneofibular ligament lie in same vertical plane. The goniometer has been moved over the specimen. *a*, Goniometer; *b*, Kirschner wire; *c*, axis rod.

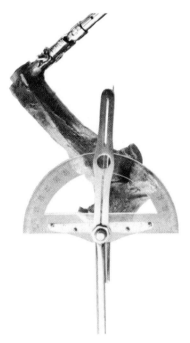

**Figure G-3.**  Top view showing goniometer and underlying specimen. The goniometer is moved until the center overlies the point of intersection of the rod and the wire. The angle between the rod and the wire is measured as the subtalar joint is moved through its full range.

the calcaneofibular ligament are viewed in a horizontal plane (Fig. G-4), it will be readily seen that they intersect posteriorly and diverge anteriorly. The reason for this arrangement is obviously the necessity for the two bony attachments of the ligament to lie close to the functional axis of the ankle at its proximal end and to the functional axis of the subtalar joint at its distal end. This requires that the ligament extend from the tip of the lateral malleolus to the lateral side of the calcaneus. To fully understand the functional behavior of the ligament during movement of both ankle and subtalar joints, it was felt necessary to establish the amount of divergence and the degree of individual variation. Therefore, the following measurements were made on 50 cadaver specimens. Utilizing the same holding apparatus, the specimen was rotated so that the ligament and subtalar axis lay in the horizontal plane. With the goniometer mounted in a horizontal plane above the specimen, the angle between the axis rod and the Kirschner wire was measured (Fig. G-4). The average angle of divergence was 31° ± 6° with a maximal value of 43° and a minimal value of 19°.

**The Angle Between the Anterior Talofibular and Calcaneofibular Ligaments.**  Since it has been shown that the axis of the subtalar joint varies in its inclination and since the calcaneofibular ligament has been demonstrated to closely parallel the axis when projected onto the sagittal plane, it appeared likely that the angle between the anterior talofibular and the calcaneofibular ligaments would show individual variations. The directions of the fibers of the two ligaments, however, are

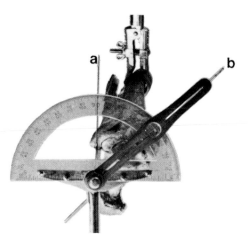

**Figure G-4.** Specimen viewed from below and oriented so that axis rod and Kirschner wire lie in same horizontal plane. The divergence of the axis rod from the wire is measured with the goniometer. *a*, Kirschner wire in calcaneofibular ligament; *b*, axis rod.

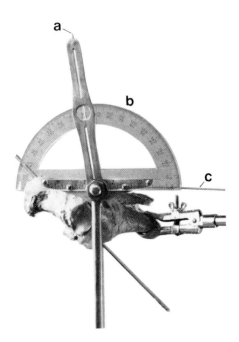

**Figure G-5.** Specimen oriented by eye so that Kirschner wires inserted into calcaneofibular and anterior talofibular ligaments lie in same horizontal plane. The goniometer has been adjusted so that one wire parallels the base of the goniometer and the other wire parallels the movable arm. *a*, Wire in anterior talofibular ligament; *b*, goniometer; *c*, wire in calcaneofibular ligament.

quite different, with the talofibular ligament coursing almost transversely and the calcaneofibular ligament running anteriorly and laterally.

The selection of a plane upon which to project and measure the angle between the two ligaments became a problem. Two planes were selected and the angle was measured in both.

The first plane was established by orienting the specimen so that the two Kirschner wires (one in the anterior talofibular ligament and the other in the calcaneofibular ligament) lay in the same horizontal plane. The goniometer, held horizontally on its own support stand, was moved over the specimen, and the projected angle between the Kirschner wires in the two ligaments was measured in the midposition of the subtalar joint and in maximal inversion and eversion of the calcaneus on the talus (Fig. G-5). The average angle between the anterior talofibular ligament and the calcaneofibular ligament measured in the midposition of the subtalar joint was 105° ± 24°. A minimal value of 75° was recorded in one specimen and a maximal value of 139° in another. With inversion and eversion of the calcaneus, the angle changed a varying amount in every specimen. On the average, the angle decreased to 93° ± 31° on inversion and increased to 113° ± 32° on eversion. No significant differences were found between the right and left sides.

The second plane selected was one that was perpendicular to the empirical axis of the ankle joint. The specimen was rotated until the 3-mm rod representing the empirical axis of the ankle joint was vertical. The angle between the wires was measured in the same manner as above. The angle measured in this plane differed from the angle measured in the sagittal plane in most specimens. It was less in 26, greater in 13, and the same in 11 specimens. The average angle was 106° ± 24°, with a range between 86 and 128°. It was surprising to find that the average values of the angles taken in the two different planes were so comparable. Furthermore, inversion and eversion of the calcaneus produced the same change in the angle. Inversion decreased the angle to 99° ± 25° and eversion increased the angle to 111° ± 26°.

# Appendix H

## Ranges of motion at the subtalar joint

This Appendix describes the techniques employed in the study on the ranges of motion in the subtalar joint. The studies were carried out on cadaver material and on living individuals.

### CADAVER STUDIES

This section reports on two independent studies done three years apart by different investigators, on two separate series of cadaver feet. The first series consisted of 47 and the second of 102 specimens. They are reported separately.

**Series I (47 Specimens).** The calcaneus and talus were removed together from cadaver feet. All soft tissues were removed except the capsular and ligamentous structures connecting the two bones. The axis of the subtalar joint was located and a stainless steel pin inserted in the usual manner (Appendix F). The calcaneus was held in a vise and the talus remained free to rotate about the empirically located axis. A protractor was mounted on and perpendicular to the stainless steel axis that protruded from the talus. A 0.5-mm stainless steel pin was drilled into the head of the talus, parallel to the plane of the protractor. The talus was rotated through its full range of possible motion and the angle of this total motion was recorded. The embalming process obviously resulted in some restriction of motion, particularly as a result of loss of elasticity in the interosseous talocalcaneal ligament. Therefore, all ligaments were carefully removed and the ranges of motion again recorded with the talus free to move on the calcaneus without the restriction of any ligamentous structures. The joint was rotated through its full range with manual pressure to keep the articulating surfaces in contact, extremes of movement being limited by osseous contact. Obviously the first series of measurements was probably less than normal whereas the second series may have demonstrated excessive motion.

The average amount of motion in the first series of measurements was 18° ± 6°, with a range of 10 to 41°. In the second series of measurements, the average was 36° ± 10°, with a range of 17 to 59°.

**Series II (102 Specimens).** The cadaver specimens utilized in the investigation of the screwlike movement between the talus and calcaneus (Appendix F) also yielded data on the range of motion at the subtalar joint. The extremes of motion were terminated when articular cartilage of the talus no longer contacted the articular surface of the posterior facet of the calcaneus.

In this series the right and left sides were recorded separately to determine whether any obvious differences would appear, but none were seen. The results are shown in Table H-1.

**Table H-1.**
**Range of Motion at Subtalar Joint**

| Subtalar Joint | No. of Specimens | Average | Range |
|---|---|---|---|
| Right | 48 | 24.7° ± 10.6° | 5–54° |
| Left | 54 | 23.2 ± 11.4 | 4–55 |
| Total | 102 | 24 ± 11 | 4–55 |

## NORMAL SUBJECTS

The total range of motion in the subtalar joint was determined in an unselected group of 50 subjects. Both right and left feet were measured, providing data on 100 feet. There were 14 men and 36 women. The age range was 22 to 62 years, with an average of 34 years. None of the subjects gave a history of fractures or sprains about the ankle or of persistent foot pain, nor were any deformities revealed on examination or any abnormalities of gait demonstrated.

The technique for measuring the range of motion was based upon the positioning of the foot and the use of a specially constructed spherical goniometer. Both the positioning of the foot and the construction and use of the goniometer require more detailed discussion.

Ideally, the motion between the talus and the calcaneus should be measured in a plane that is at a right angle to the axis of rotation. However, the position of the axis has been shown to be variable and in the living can only be roughly estimated. An attempt was made to achieve measurements that were as accurate as possible by employing a specially constructed spherical goniometer and utilizing "set" positions of the leg and foot.

**Spherical Goniometer.** A glass sphere, 5 cm in diameter, was the basic element of the goniometer. It was filled with water and sealed, except for a tiny air bubble with a diameter of approximately 2 mm (Fig. H-1). This provided a type of level in which the bubble remained always in a vertical position over the center of the sphere, no matter how the sphere the tilted or rotated. A movable scale was fitted over the sphere and glued to two sectors of a sphere of clear plastic. This arrangement permitted the scale to be moved while always lying in a meridian of the spherical level. When used, the spherical goniometer was fixed to a laminated plastic heel cup (Fig. H-2A) or a molded plastic platform for application to the dorsum of the foot (Fig. H-2B). The methods of application of the goniometers to the foot are shown in Figure H-3, *A* and *B*.

**Positioning of the Foot.** To assure that the measurements obtained from the spherical goniometer would be reasonably accurate, the axis of the subtalar joint should be as nearly horizontal as possible. To achieve this, two positions of the leg and foot were utilized. The subject first was placed prone and the knee flexed to 135°, the foot being kept at a right angle to the lower leg. Since the average inclination of the axis is around 45°, this position places the axis approximately in a horizontal plane. Knee flexion relaxed the gastrocnemius and obviated any restrictive influence that it might exert on the free movement of the subtalar joint. The second position consisted of having the subject sit on the edge of the examining table with the knee flexed to

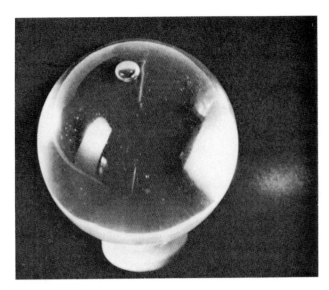

**Figure H-1.** Basic element of spherical goniometer. A glass sphere is filled with water and sealed. A small bubble of air remains that can move along any great circle pathway within the sphere and always remain vertical to the center of the sphere no matter what rotational displacement occurs.

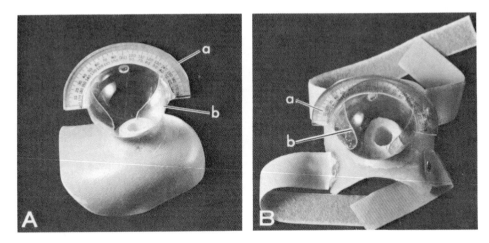

**Figure H-2.** Completely assembled spherical goniometers for determination of ranges of motion in subtalar joints. *a*, Scales glued to two sectors of sphere (*b*). These scales can be moved to overlie any pathway of travel of the bubble. **A**, Spherical goniometer glued to laminated heel cup. **B**, Spherical goniometer glued to molded laminated platform for application to dorsum of foot. Straps of Velcro have been provided for firm fixation of the platform to the foot.

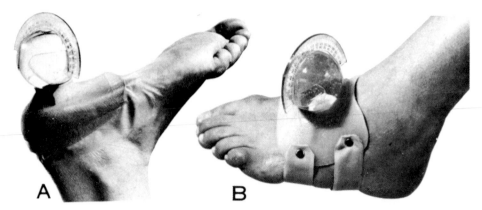

**Figure H-3.** Attachment of goniometers to foot. **A,** Laminated heel cup firmly taped to skin of heel. **B,** Laminated plastic platform held rigidly in place on dorsum of foot by means of two straps of Velcro.

90°. The foot was passively plantar flexed to approximately 45°. This maneuver again places the average subtalar axis in approximately a horizontal plane (Fig. H-4).

## RATIONALE AND USE OF THE SPHERICAL GONIOMETER

A more detailed exposition of the principles that led to the development and use of the spherical goniometer appears necessary. This will be attempted by employing both written descriptions and drawings. The presentation will be sequential, starting with basic concepts and progressing to the practical application of the device.

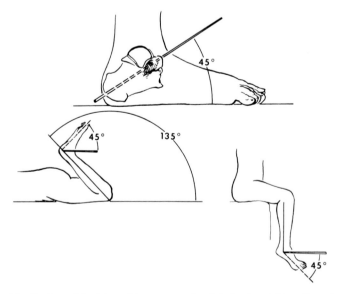

**Figure H-4.** Positioning of foot to achieve approximately horizontal location of subtalar axis. Two positions are available, achieved either by flexion of the knee to 135° with the subject prone or by plantar flexion of the foot to 45° with the subject sitting.

The use of gravity to establish one arm of the angle to be measured accomplished two purposes. It obviated the need to locate precisely the axis of rotation, and the goniometer could be located at any distance from the axis. This is demonstrated in the sketch with the use of plumb bobs (Fig. H-5). A spherical level acts in the same manner as does a plumb bob.

The accuracy of the measurement of the rotation obviously depends upon the axis remaining in a horizontal plane. This is attempted by placing the subject in first one and then the other of the two positions (see Fig. H-4). Unfortunately it can not be determined whether in any individual the positioning of the foot in space assures that the axis is precisely horizontal. The anthropometric studies indicate that the axis may vary 20° on either side of the mean of 42°. In both situations, the angle measured will be less than the actual amount of rotation. This decrease in the measured angle will vary as the cosine of the angle of deviation of the axis from the horizontal.

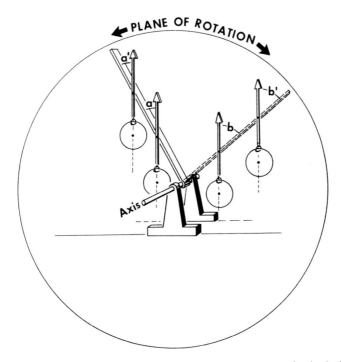

**Figure H-5.** Diagrammatic demonstration of principle underlying use of spherical goniometer. Plumb bobs have been mounted at varying distances on arms extending from a horizontal axis. Since the axis is horizontal and the plumb bobs are always vertical, the angles will remain equal no matter how far removed from the axis of rotation ($<a = <a'$ and $<b = <b'$). The *circle* at the bottom of each pendulum represents the spherical goniometer. The sphere is filled with fluid except for a small bubble, which will always align itself vertically with the center of the sphere and thus behave in a manner similar to that of a plumb bob. Obviously, because of its spherical construction, the bubble is free to move in several planes, making it more versatile than a plumb bob, which records accurately in only one plane. After application of the spherical goniometer to the foot, the pathway of the bubble along an arc of a great circle is noted and a movable scale is aligned to the path of travel.

Reference to trigonometric tables indicates that the maximal error involved is probably less than 10%.

It should be noted that the axis of the subtalar joint also varies in the transverse plane, being inclined medially from the midline of the foot from 4 to 48°. The spherical goniometer automatically accommodates this variation with rotation. The bubble will move through an arc of a great circle that is perpendicular to the axis of motion. All that is necessary is to adjust the movable scale over the sphere so that it lies in the plane of travel of the bubble. The procedure employed in measuring the range of motion in the subtalar joint with the spherical goniometer was as follows.

1. The subject was placed prone with the knee flexed to 135° and the foot held at a right angle to the leg.
2. A snugly fitting heel cup carrying the spherical goniometer was taped securely to the heel of the subject.
3. The forefoot was maximally inverted and everted passively by the examiner. The rotatory forces were applied to the forefoot in such a way as not to cause any displacement of the heel cup on the heel. The path of the bubble was noted and the scale was moved so as to lie over the path of travel of the bubble. The total angular movement was noted and recorded (Fig. H-6).
4. The subject was next asked to sit on the edge of the table with the knee flexed to 90° and the foot plantar flexed approximately 45°. A second goniometer was taped to the dorsum of the foot.
5. By grasping the heel, the examiner forcibly inverted and everted the heel. The remainder of the foot followed the displacement of the heel passively (Fig. H-7).

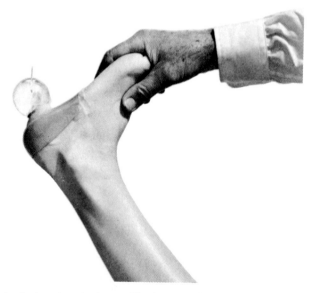

**Figure H-6.** Spherical goniometer in use. The heel cup carrying the goniometer has been taped securely to the heel. With the leg stabilized by one hand of the examiner, the other hand inverts and everts the forefoot while maintaining the foot at a right angle to the leg. The excursion of the bubble is measured on the circular scale.

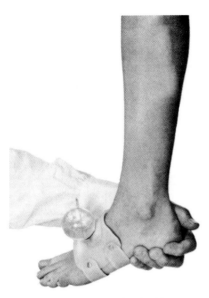

**Figure H-7.** Motion in subtalar joint being checked by measuring motion of forefoot. The spherical goniometer has been strapped to the foot. The examiner rotates the heel, and the excursion of the bubble is measured on the circular scale.

6. The movement of the bubble was again noted, and the scale was adjusted to overlie the path of the bubble.
7. The angular displacement with passive maximal inversion and eversion of the heel was noted and recorded.

   Differences in measurements as recorded from heel and forefoot occurred in most subjects, but they rarely exceeded 10°. The range of motion measured with the goniometer on the heel tended to be greater than the motion recorded with the goniometer on the dorsum of the foot. Histograms of the measurements revealed nearly perfect distribution curves.

   The average range of motion with the goniometer on the heel was 44° ± 7°, with a range of 24 to 65°. The average range of motion with the goniometer on the dorsum of the foot was 36° ± 8°, with a range of 20 to 50°. If the two measurements are combined, the average range of motion is approximately 40°, with a range of 20 to 62°. Scatter diagrams indicated no correlation between ranges of motion and sex or age in this series.

   Attention is directed to the differences in the values for the average amount of motion in the subtalar joint obtained from the cadaver studies as compared with those in the living. The cadaver studies yielded averages that are approximately half as large as those calculated from measurements on the living. Several explanations for these differences are possible. A review of the data from each of the studies reveals that the maximal amounts of motion recorded in all three studies were comparable (55, 59, and 65°). However, in the cadaver studies, the minimal amount of movement was far less than in the living. Recorded measurements of only a few degrees of motion were frequent in the cadaver specimens, while the minimal amount of motion recorded in the living was 20°. The presence of smaller measurements would naturally tend to lower the average value of the range of motion in the cadaver series. These smaller measurements on the amount of motion in the cadaver might have resulted from embalming, but conversely, the motion measured on the living might have been excessive. Several factors might be mentioned that could contribute to abnormally large measurements as recorded in the living. The joints were passively moved by the investigator and the articular surfaces were not under compression, thus possibly permitting abnormal separation of the joint surfaces at the extremes of movement. The goniometer could not be fixed rigidly to the bony structures, and the displacement of the goniometer was necessarily carried out through soft tissues. Therefore, movement in joints other than the subtalar joint may have occurred. Assuming that the true value for the average range of motion in the subtalar joint lies somewhere between 24 and 44°, this amount of motion is two to three times that commonly quoted in the literature.

# Index